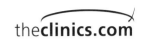

DENTAL CLINICS

OF NORTH AMERICA

Geriatrics: Contemporary and
Future Concerns

GUEST EDITOR
Roseann Mulligan, DDS, MS

D1474873

April 2005 • Volume 49 • Number 2

SAUNDERS

An Imprint of Elsevier, Inc.
PHILADELPHIA LONDON TORONTO MONTREAL SYDNEY TOKYO

W.B. SAUNDERS COMPANY
A Division of Elsevier Inc.

The Curtis Center • Independence Square West • Philadelphia, Pennsylvania 19106

http://www.dental.theclinics.com

THE DENTAL CLINICS OF NORTH AMERICA	**Volume 49, Number 2**
April 2005	**ISSN 0011-8532**
Editor: John Vassallo	**ISBN 1-4160-2820-X**

The ideas and opinions expressed in *The Dental Clinics of North America* do not necessarily reflect those of the Publisher. The Publisher does not assume any responsibility for any injury and/or damage to persons or property arising out of or related to any use of the material contained in this periodical. The reader is advised to check the appropriate medical literature and the product information currently provided by the manufacturer of each drug to be administered to verify the dosage, the method and duration of administration, or contraindications. It is the responsibility of the treating physician or other health care professional, relying on independent experience and knowledge of the patient, to determine drug dosages and the best treatment for the patient. Mention of any product in this issue should not be construed as endorsement by the contributors, editors, or the Publisher of the product or manufacturers' claims.

The Dental Clinics of North America (ISSN 0011-8532) is published quarterly by W.B. Saunders Company. Corporate and Editorial Offices: The Curtis Center, Independence Square West, Philadelphia, PA 19106-3399. Accounting and circulation offices: 6277 Sea Harbor Drive, Orlando, FL 32887-4800. Periodicals postage paid at Orlando, FL 32862, and additional mailing offices. Subscription prices are $150.00 per year (US individuals), $242.00 per year (US institutions), $181.00 per year (Canadian individuals), $299.00 per year (Canadian institutions), $75.00 per year (US students/residents), $205.00 per year (foreign individuals), and $299.00 per year (foreign institutions) and $103.00 (Canadian and foreign students/residents). Foreign air speed delivery is included in all *Clinics* subscription prices. All prices are subject to change without notice. POSTMASTER: Send address changes to *The Dental Clinics of North America*, W.B. Saunders Company, Periodicals Fulfillment, Orlando, FL 32887-4800. **Customer Service: 1-800-654-2452 (US). From outside of the US, call 1-407-345-4000.**

The Dental Clinics of North America is covered in *Index Medicus, Current Contents/Clinical Medicine, ISI/BIOMED and Clinahl.*

Printed in the United States of America.

GUEST EDITOR

ROSEANN MULLIGAN, DDS, MS, Professor, Schools of Dentistry and Gerontology; and Associate Dean for Community Health Programs, School of Dentistry, University of Southern California, Los Angeles, California

CONTRIBUTORS

JANE C. ATKINSON, DDS, Professor and Chair, Comprehensive Care and Therapeutics, University of Maryland Dental School, Baltimore, Maryland

JACK S. BROUSSARD, Jr, DDS, G. Donald Montgomery Professorship in Dentistry, Associate Professor, Clinical Dentistry, Division of Primary Care; and Director, University of Southern California Oral Health Center, University of Southern California, School of Dentistry, Los Angeles, California

GLENN T. CLARK, DDS, MS, Professor and Director, Orofacial Pain and Oral Medicine Center; and Division of Diagnostic Sciences, University of Southern California, School of Dentistry, Los Angeles, California

SAMUEL C. DURSO, MD, AGSF, Associate Professor of Medicine; Clinical Director; and Director of Education, Division of Geriatric Medicine and Gerontology, Johns Hopkins University School of Medicine, Baltimore, Maryland

VERONICA A. GREENE, DDS, MPH, Assistant Professor, Department of Clinical Dentistry, University of Southern California School of Dentistry, Los Angeles, California

MARGARET GRISIUS, DMD, Consultant, Gene Therapy and Therapeutics Branch, National Institute of Dental and Craniofacial Research, Bethesda, Maryland

JIWON KIM, PharmD, Assistant Professor, Clinical Pharmacy, University of Southern California, School of Pharmacy, Los Angeles, California

ANA C. LOTAIF, DDS, MS, Assistant Professor and Clinical Manager, Orofacial Pain and Oral Medicine Center; and Division of Diagnostic Sciences, University of Southern California, School of Dentistry, Los Angeles, California

MICHAEL I. MacENTEE, LDS(I), Dip Prosth, FRCD(C), PhD, Faculty of Dentistry, University of British Columbia, Vancouver, British Columbia, Canada

DANIEL MALAMUD, PhD, Professor, Department of Biochemistry, School of Dental Medicine, University of Pennsylvania, Philadelphia, Pennsylvania

WARD MASSEY, BDS, PhD, Assistant Professor, Restorative Dentistry and Biomaterials Science, Harvard School of Dental Medicine, Boston, Massachusetts

CYRIL MEYEROWITZ, BDS, MS, Professor and Chair, Eastman Department of Dentistry, University of Rochester; and Director, Eastman Dental Center, Rochester, New York

HAJIME MINAKUCHI, DDS, PhD, Visiting Research Scholar, Orofacial Pain and Oral Medicine Center; and Division of Diagnostic Sciences, University of Southern California, School of Dentistry, Los Angeles, California

ROSEANN MULLIGAN, DDS, MS, Professor, Schools of Dentistry and Gerontology; and Associate Dean for Community Health Programs, School of Dentistry, University of Southern California, Los Angeles, California

G. RUTGER PERSSON, DDS, PhD (Odont Dr), Professor, Department of Periodontology and Fixed Prosthodontics, Faculty of Medicine, University of Berne, Berne, Switzerland; and Department of Periodontics, Department of Oral Medicine, School of Dentistry, University of Washington, Seattle, Washington

RIGMOR E. PERSSON, DDS, MSD, Research Associate Professor, Department of Periodontology and Fixed Prosthodontics, Faculty of Medicine, University of Berne, Berne, Switzerland; and Department of Oral Medicine, School of Dentistry, University of Washington, Seattle, Washington

RALPH H. SAUNDERS, Jr, DDS, MS, Associate Professor, Eastman Department of Dentistry, University of Rochester; and Director of Dental Service, Monroe Community Hospital, Rochester, New York

YOLANDA ANN SLAUGHTER, DDS, MPH, Assistant Professor, Department of Preventive and Restorative Sciences, School of Dental Medicine, University of Pennsylvania, Philadelphia, Pennsylvania

STEPHEN SOBEL, DDS, Associate Professor of Clinical Dentistry, Division of Diagnostic Sciences, School of Dentistry, University of Southern California, Los Angeles, California

BRADLEY R. WILLIAMS, PharmD, FASCP, CGP, Associate Professor, Clinical Pharmacy and Clinical Gerontology, University of Southern California, School of Pharmacy, Los Angeles, California

JANET A. YELLOWITZ, DMD, MPH, Associate Professor and Director of Geriatric Dentistry, University of Maryland, Baltimore College of Dental Surgery, Department of Health Promotion and Policy, Baltimore, Maryland

CONTENTS

The increasing population of older subjects with dental care needs
will become a major challenge to our society and its care providers.
To manage the health care needs of the elderly, a coordination between medical and dental care providers will become necessary.
From the dental perspective, it is important to develop skills in
the risk assessment of older patients. Such risk assessment of older
subjects should take an approach that is holistic and focused on the
reduction of the infectious burden and the improvement of self-
efficacy.

Dental caries is one of the most significant health problems facing
older adults. More than half of the elderly who are dentate are affected with either coronal or root caries, and caries is the primary
cause of tooth loss in this population. New materials and techniques are emerging to help with geriatric preventive and restorative needs, but ongoing vigilance for caries will be required in this
population, which is experiencing increased longevity and tooth
retention.

Salivary gland hypofunction and complaints of xerostomia are
common in elderly patients, irrespective of their living situation.

Medication use is frequently related to dry mouth symptoms and reductions in salivary flow rates. Patients with reduced salivary flow are at increased risk for caries, oral fungal infections, swallowing problems, and diminished or altered taste. Oral health care providers should institute aggressive preventive measures and recommend palliative care for patients with significant reduction in salivary gland function. The systemic agents pilocarpine and cevimeline may help selected patients. Selective use of fluoride-releasing restorative materials and conservative treatment plans are recommended for this patient group.

Temporomandibular joint (TMJ) dysfunction is often believed to be a young person's malady. However, geriatric patients also present with clinical findings of TMJ clicking, locking, crepitation, limited opening, and pain. With our aging population and the high prevalence of rheumatic and musculoskeletal diseases in the elderly, it is important to understand the etiopathogenesis, clinical presentation, and management of derangement, rheumatoid arthritis, and osteoarthritis of the TMJ. Although arthritis of the TMJ usually causes only mild-to-moderate dysfunction in older patients, they present challenges related to medication use and comorbidity. This article presents the most recent understanding and therapeutic protocols for patient diagnosis and management.

Many orofacial pain conditions occur in the elderly. Specifically, this article reviews the prevalence of general and orofacial-related pain in the elderly. The authors also describe and discuss the likely disorders and diseases that produce facial pain and burning pain in the mouth. They do not cover jaw joint pain, oral sores, or ulceration-induced pain, as these conditions are better discussed in the context of arthritis and oral pathologies of the mouth. The authors discuss oral motor disorders, myogenous pain, vascular pain, headaches, trigeminal neuralgia, trigeminal neuropathic disease, postherpetic neuralgia, burning mouth syndrome, and occlusal dysesthesia.

The elderly represent approximately 12.4% of the general population (2000 Census), yet their health care expenditure and consumption represent 14% of the total (2003). Although 10% of the elderly had no medical insurance in 2000, 78% had no dental insurance. Elderly Americans' burden of medical care overuse is worsened by their out-of-pocket expenses for oral health, because this is usually not a covered benefit. In underserved communities, the management of the oral health and dental care needs of older Americans approaches negligence.

Comprehensive health care of the geriatric patient requires thoughtful communication and coordination of services. Unlike young adults, older patients are likely to be frail, have multiple chronic conditions, and experience disability. Hence they are more likely to depend on others for help and to see a variety of health professionals at different sites. This complexity demands that health care professionals consider their care not in isolation, but as part of a team. They must ensure that other members of the team are kept informed and are consulted as appropriate to ensure safe and effective care. Accomplishing this goal requires being acquainted with the usual care providers, the necessary information for sharing, and the most effective communication methods within the team.

As the population ages, dental and other health care providers will be working with more older adults (and their family members) with changing cognitive status than ever before in history. The intent of this article is to review common cognitive changes in older adults that will undoubtedly be seen in dental practices. Knowledge of the common signs and symptoms of age-related cognitive changes provides a basis on which to identify individuals with undiagnosed cognitive changes. This article reviews the relationship between cognitive function, aging, and dementia (specifically, mild cognitive impairment and Alzheimer's disease), the role of the dental team in recognizing these conditions, and issues related to obtaining informed consent from cognitively impaired patients.

Older adults consume more medications than any other segment of the population. Increasing lifespan means that more people will live into old age, frequently with disabilities and conditions managed by medications. Age-associated physiologic changes, medication use patterns, and adverse drug effects and interactions place the older adult at high risk for medication-related problems. Older adults living in institutions, those with complex medical problems, and those who do not adhere to medication regimens are at highest risk for negative health outcomes from medication mishaps. Dentists must be able to identify older adults who are susceptible to adverse drug events and to recognize which medications are most likely to precipitate problems.

FORTHCOMING ISSUES

RECENT ISSUES

GOAL STATEMENT
The goal of the *Dental Clinics of North America* is to keep practicing dentists up to date with current clinical practice in dentistry by providing timely articles reviewing the state of the art in dental care.

ACCREDITATION
The *Dental Clinics of North America* are planned and implemented in accordance with the ADA CERP Recognition Standards and Procedures through the joint sponsorship with Virginia Commonwealth University, School of Dentistry Office of Continuing Education, the University of Virginia School of Medicine, and W.B. Saunders Company.

Virginia Commonwealth University, School of Dentistry is designated as an ADA CERP Recognized Provider. Virginia Commonwealth University, School of Dentistry is a Recognized Academy of General Dentistry Program Provider, Code 0216.

Dentists participating in this learning activity may earn up to 15 ADA CERP credits per issue or a maximum of 60 credits per year. Credits awarded may not apply toward license renewal in all states. It is the responsibility of each participant to verify the requirements of their state licensing board.

ADA CERP credit can be earned by reading the text material, taking the examination online at *http://www.theclinics.com/home/cme*, and completing the evaluation. Each test question must be answered correctly; you will have the opportunity to retake any questions answered incorrectly. Following successful completion of the test and the evaluation, you may print your certificate.

FACULTY DISCLOSURE
The University of Virginia School of Medicine is accredited by the Accreditation Council for Continuing Medical Education (ACCME) to provide continuing medical education for physicians.

As a provider accredited by the Accreditation Council for Continuing Medical Education (ACCME), the Office of Continuing Medical Education of the University of Virginia School of Medicine must ensure balance, independence, objectivity, and scientific rigor in all its individually sponsored or jointly sponsored educational activities. All authors/editors participating in a sponsored activity are expected to disclose to the readers any significant financial interest or other relationship (1) with the manufacturer(s) of any commercial product(s) and/or provider(s) of commercial services discussed in an educational presentation and (2) with any commercial supporters of the activity (significant financial interest or other relationship can include such things as grants or research support, employee, consultant, stock holder, member of speakers bureau, etc.). The intent of this disclosure is not to prevent authors/editors with a significant financial or other relationship from writing an article, but rather to provide readers with information on which they can make their own judgments. It remains for the readers to determine whether the author's/editor's interest or relationships may influence the article with regard to exposition or conclusion.

The authors/editors listed below have identified no professional or financial affiliations related to the articles:
Jack S. Broussard, Jr, DDS; Samuel C. Durso, MD; Veronica A. Greene, DDS, MPH; Jiwon Kim, PharmD; Michael I. MacEntee, LDS(I), Dip Prosth, FRCD(C), PhD; Daniel Malamud, PhD; Ward Massey, BDS, PhD; Cyril Meyerowitz, BDS, MS; Roseann Mulligan, DDS, MS; G. Rutger Persson, DDS, PhD; Rigmor E. Persson, DDS, MSD; Ralph H. Saunders, Jr, DDS, MS; Yolanda Ann Slaughter, DDS, MPH; Stephen Sobel, DDS; John Vassallo, Acquisitions Editor; Bradley R. Williams, PharmD, FASCP, CGP; and Janet A. Yellowitz, DMD, MPH.

Disclosure of discussion of non-FDA approved uses for pharmaceutical products and/or medical devices:
The University of Virginia School of Medicine, as an ACCME provider, requires that all authors/editors identify and disclose any "off label" uses for pharmaceutical products and/or for medical devices. The University of Virginia School of Medicine recommends that each reader fully review all the available data on new products or procedures prior to instituting them with patients.

All authors/editors who provided disclosures will not be discussing any off-label uses except:
Roseann Mulligan, DDS, MS and Stephen Sobel, DDS will discuss the use of Etidronate and Pamidronate for osteoporosis.

The authors/editors listed below have not provided disclosure or off-label information:
Jane C. Atkinson, DDS; Glenn T. Clark, DDS, MS; Margaret Grisius, DMD; and Ana C. Lotaif, DDS, MS; and Hajime Minakuchi, DDS, PhD.

TO ENROLL
To enroll in the Dental Clinics of North America Continuing Medical Education program, call customer service at 1-800-654-2452 or sign up online at *http://www.theclinics.com/home/cme*. The CME program is available to subscribers for an additional annual fee of $79.95.

THE DENTAL
CLINICS
OF NORTH AMERICA

Dent Clin N Am 49 (2005) xi–xiii

Preface

Geriatrics: Contemporary and Future Concerns

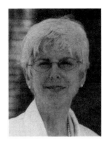

Roseann Mulligan, DDS, MS
Guest Editor

The explosion in size of the elderly population in this country and throughout the world's developing countries is a phenomenon that is now widely recognized as being in its infancy. US Census predictions that the population aged 65 years and over will double from the 35 million of 2000 to 69 million by 2030 are well established. As more people are becoming elderly, they are entering these years with heightened oral health expectations and are seeking care in much greater numbers than did similarly aged cohorts of previous generations. What are the current issues and most recent findings with regard to care of elderly patients, and what might the future hold in terms of diagnostics and health issues for this population? This issue sets out to address these questions. At the same time, it is important to understand that not all elderly people are at a similar level of oral health care awareness, recognition of need, or access to services. The 2000 *Surgeon General's Report on Oral Health in America* (available at http://www2. nidcr.nih.gov/sgr/sgrohweb/welcome.htm) clearly demonstrated that minority populations in this country have poor oral health, and this is true of the minority elderly as well. In this issue, Dr. Veronica Greene provides an update on the status of the oral health of elderly minority populations.

Today's elders are affected by caries, periodontal disease, diminished salivary function, orofacial pain, and arthritis of the temporomandibular joint. Rigmor E. Persson and G. Rutger Persson discuss chronic periodontitis in the elderly, the dearth of periodontal research focused on the truly elderly, and the systemic implications of periodontal disease for this

doi:10.1016/j.cden.2004.11.002   *dental.theclinics.com*

population. Ralph H. Saunders and Cyril Meyerowitz consider the high prevalence of both coronal and root caries and current and future prevention and management methods. Jane C. Atkinson, Margie Grisius, and Ward Massey cover the conditions of salivary hypofunction and xerostomia, which can have a contributory role in the evolution of carious lesions; they also discuss the prevention and treatment modifications required to manage these conditions and their impact on each other. The clinical presentation and management of the most common temporomandibular joint conditions, including rheumatoid arthritis, osteoarthritis, and derangement, are the foci of the article by Jack S. Broussard. Glenn T. Clark, Hajime Minakuchi, and Ana C. Lotaif consider the clinical recognition and treatment of chronic orofacial pain, sensory disorders, and dyskinesias, which are found with some frequency in this population.

Many conditions covered in these papers will be managed by using medications that in and of themselves may be problematic for elderly patients or that may cause negative interactions when combined with medications prescribed by the dentist. Bradley R. Williams and Jiwon Kim remind us of medication usage patterns in the elderly, the adverse reactions that occur in this age group, and the dentist's role in recognizing patients and medications that are more likely to be at risk for negative outcomes.

As greater numbers of elders and their families seek dental care, there will be many who have developed chronic systemic conditions. Consultations with other health care providers and interdisciplinary teamwork will become crucial to managing the elderly patient's treatment. Samuel C. Durso discusses the interaction and consultation among the formal and informal members of the health care team that is needed to provide safe, effective, and appropriate care to the elderly patient.

With increasing age, the likelihood of cognitive decline also increases. Janet A. Yellowitz addresses this concern in her paper on cognitive functioning, how to recognize declines, and the impact these declines could have on ethical, legal, and care delivery issues.

As the older population expands, more elderly people will become residents of long-term care facilities. Michael I. MacEntee discusses the exceptional oral health findings related to this population and the present caregiving and management challenges. He proposes questions that need to be addressed in future studies if we are to improve the oral health of this vulnerable group.

To round out this issue, two articles discuss important developments in dentistry that are likely to have a proportionally greater impact on the elderly. The article by Yolanda Ann Slaughter and Daniel Malamud discusses the field of oral diagnostics and the role it may play in risk assessment, diagnosis of oral disease, and therapeutic drug monitoring for oral and systemic disease. The authors outline the benefits of oral sampling over blood or urine sampling. The article by Roseann Mulligan and Stephen Sobel addresses the all-important issue of osteoporosis, a condition that is increasingly present with aging and causes bone fractures in one of every two women and one of every four men. Osteoporosis may be implicated in periodontal disease and may play a role in implant success; in the future, it may be routinely diagnosable through dental radiographs.

In summary, it has been our goal in this issue to provide readers with an update on the current issues in geriatric dentistry related to diagnosis and management of the most commonly occurring conditions. We have also described clinical concerns where the definitive answers are not yet available and for which we need additional research. Finally, we have given readers a glimpse of new diagnostic methods that may await the geriatric dentist of the future.

I offer thanks to all the contributors to this issue for working so diligently to bring readers the most up-to-date information.

Roseann Mulligan, DDS, MS
University of Southern California
School of Dentistry
925 West 34th Street
Los Angeles, CA 90089-0641, USA

E-mail address: mulligan@usc.edu

ELSEVIER
SAUNDERS

Dent Clin N Am 49 (2005) 279–292

THE DENTAL
CLINICS
OF NORTH AMERICA

The Elderly at Risk for Periodontitis and Systemic Diseases

Rigmor E. Persson, DDS, MSD[a,b,*],
G. Rutger Persson, DDS, PhD(Odont Dr)[a,c]

[a]*Department of Periodontology and Fixed Prosthodontics,
University of Berne, Freiburgstrasse 7, CH 3010 Berne, Switzerland*
[b]*Department of Oral Medicine, School of Dentistry, University of Washington,
Box 356370, Seattle, WA 98195-6370, USA*
[c]*Department of Periodontics, School of Dentistry, University of Washington,
D-570 Health Sciences Center, Seattle, WA 98195, USA*

The challenges to society of managing the services and well being of older subjects will consume an increasingly larger proportion of human and financial resources. From a macroeconomic perspective, the United States could afford to let health spending grow more rapidly than the overall gross domestic product, but only by pricing low-income Americans out of health care [1]. This development would specifically affect older subjects, because most retirees choose not to include dental insurance in their health insurance plans. Periodontitis has an infectious etiology. The oral infectious burden resulting from periodontitis may aggravate systemic health in the elderly.

Both "periodontal disease" and "elderly" are terms that lack firm definitions. The definition of "elderly" is routinely based on chronologic age rather than on biologic age. Preferably, the biologic age should define whether an individual is elderly. Nevertheless, three groups of older subjects are often identified based on chronologic age: (1) young-old (65–74 years), (2) old-old (75–84 years), and (3) oldest old (>85 years). The current periodontal literature is insufficient to describe how the prevalence and severity of periodontitis are distributed among these three defined groups of elderly people.

* Corresponding author. Department of Oral Medicine, Box 356370, School of Dentistry, University of Washington, Seattle, WA 98195-6370.
E-mail address: rigmor@u.washington.edu (R.E. Persson).

0011-8532/05/$ - see front matter © 2005 Elsevier Inc. All rights reserved.
doi:10.1016/j.cden.2004.10.006
dental.theclinics.com

The Surgeon General's Report on Oral Health in America [2] includes specific concerns about periodontal conditions in older Americans. The report projected that more than 20% of older people have periodontitis, that men are more often affected than women, and that older people with low income are at greater risk. In Europe and North America, the proportion of older people in society is growing rapidly. Major concerns have been raised about how these people will be cared for. Between 2001 and 2002, the United States' national health expenditures increased by 9.3%, 5% faster than the growth of the national economy [3]. It is likely that medical care will consume most of these resources. The questions of whether periodontal care support is sufficient to manage the periodontal treatment needs of the elderly and whether the treatment modalities are appropriate and available from a cost perspective are currently not well surveyed. In fact, there is a trend in periodontal therapy toward aesthetic dentistry, such as papilla preservation surgery, and toward dental implants. Both approaches may be of little relevance to the elderly and their periodontal treatment needs, as well as too expensive.

The recent discoveries that have resulted in the development of periodontal medicine as a subdiscipline in periodontology also indicate that having periodontitis may be an indicator of risk for or subclinical coexistence with other diseases. Dentists should therefore develop knowledge and skills in identifying older subjects at risk for other diseases, with a focus on infectious and chronic inflammatory-driven conditions. This proposal does not necessarily mean that dentists should diagnose medical conditions, but rather that they should refer subjects who meet specific risk profiles to physicians for further evaluation. This measure may be especially prudent in patients who plan to have invasive, extensive, and expensive dental treatments.

At the 1999 World Workshop in Periodontology, a revised diagnostic classification system was developed [4]. The new classification system replaced the previously commonly used term "adult periodontitis" with the new term "chronic periodontitis." The term "chronic periodontitis" was adopted at the workshop because it was perceived that periodontal disease can occur at any age and be found both in the primary and secondary dentition. Similarly, the previously used diagnostic terms "localized juvenile periodontitis," "early onset periodontitis," and "rapidly progressive periodontitis" were replaced by the new term "aggressive periodontitis." Both chronic and aggressive periodontitis can have localized (ie, less than 30% of teeth/surfaces affected) or generalized patterns of severity. These changes in terminology removed previous perceptions of age-related periodontal disease patterns. Under the new paradigm, there should be no differences between the etiology or pathogenesis of periodontitis in older subjects and younger subjects. In the present report on periodontal disease in the elderly, periodontal disease will be considered only as chronic periodontitis. No reports on aggressive periodontitis in the elderly currently exist.

A Medline (PubMed) search on May 18th, 2004 yielded 303 published documents using the search term "early onset periodontitis," 420 published reports using the search term "localized juvenile periodontitis," 258 reports for the term "rapidly progressive periodontitis," and 186 documents for "aggressive periodontitis." Notwithstanding, several documents might have been listed under one or more of these search terms. In contrast, a similar search using the term "periodontitis and older subjects" resulted in 65 published studies, and "periodontitis and elderly subjects" produced 486 reports. However, few of these studies specifically reported on periodontal conditions or outcomes of therapy in subjects 65 years of age or older.

These studies tend to display an enormous heterogeneity in the definitions of "older" or "elderly." Subjects aged 65 or older were excluded from participation in the vast majority of studies on periodontal therapies, including most of the classic studies on surgical and nonsurgical therapies [5]. Furthermore, none of the studies reported on treatment efficacy at the subject level. Almost all periodontal intervention studies performed between 1980 and 1995 only included subjects who were younger than 60 years. When such studies included older subjects, they never provided data on specific outcomes of periodontal treatments in this older cohort. It appears to have been taken for granted that the causes, pathogenesis, and progression of periodontitis in older subjects do not differ from those in younger adults and that, consequently, routine periodontal treatment outcomes should not differ by age. The same can be said of recent studies on the outcome of dental implant treatments. Few studies report oral implant success outcomes in older subjects.

Prevalence of periodontitis and impact of tooth loss in older subjects

A major problem in periodontal research is the lack of agreement on what constitutes periodontitis and severity of periodontitis. The current classification system for periodontitis (briefly discussed earlier) has either not been used or used with a wide range of different cut-off levels (ie, number of sites with probing depth or clinical attachment loss >2 mm). It is hence difficult to assess and compare data on the prevalence of periodontitis over time and between different regions or countries from one study to another. In addition, different dental treatment paradigms over the last 50 years have resulted in tooth extractions' being attributable partly to dental disease severity, partly to insurance benefits, but also to the more liberal attitude toward extraction in the past.

Midbuccal or midlingual gingival recession is common in many subjects and is often a consequence of tooth-brush trauma. In older subjects, however, midbuccal and midlingual gingival recession are accompanied by interproximal recession. In younger subjects, a hyperinflammatory response to infection results in edema and pseudopocketing, possibly resulting in the recording of increased pocket probing depth. In older subjects, it appears that interproximal recession and loss of attachment and alveolar bone run parallel, resulting in destruction of the periodontium in the absence of increased probing depth [6]. Notably, studies have shown that subjects with diabetes mellitus are at greater risk for clinical attachment loss, which is accompanied by an increase in gingival recession [7].

Since the mid-1960s, several studies have demonstrated a decrease in the prevalence and severity of periodontitis. However, many currently older people were young adults in the 1950s and 1960s and might have established periodontal disease at that time. Only those in the generation who remain dentate are of concern in more recent epidemiologic studies. These constitute subjects who either (1) were resistant to periodontitis, (2) received successful periodontal therapy, (3) received partially successful periodontal therapy, or (4) have periodontitis because they either were therapy-resistant or never sought care. Because tooth loss results from many factors, it is impossible to determine whether teeth were extracted as a result of periodontitis. It would therefore be difficult to assess how many subjects who were born between, for instance, 1910 and 1915 and are currently living are susceptible to periodontitis. It is easier to account for diseases such as cardiovascular disease, which result in death as an indisputable outcome measure.

Few epidemiologic studies have included older individuals. The National Health and Nutrition Examination Survey (NHANES) III study has suggested that the prevalence and severity of periodontitis increase with advancing age [8]. One study conducted among older Japanese (N= 761) demonstrated that a large majority (97%) had evidence of attachment loss and they had lost an average of three teeth [9]. The same study also demonstrated that men had more evidence of periodontitis than women and that periodontitis was more prevalent in subjects older than 80 years, especially in those with fewer than 19 remaining teeth. However the study also indicated that subjects with only nine or fewer remaining teeth had less evidence of periodontitis than those with more teeth. This finding suggests that these subjects had received therapy with selective extractions of teeth affected by periodontitis. A study of older subjects in Pomerania, Germany has confirmed that tooth loss is predominantly an effect of caries and not periodontitis [10]. Thus, the cause of tooth loss remains a difficult problem to resolve in periodontal epidemiologic studies.

Studies have shown that tooth loss in very old subjects (≥80 years) can have a significant impact not only on chewing abilities but also on general physical abilities [11]. A Norwegian study finding that approximately 30% of subjects older than 80 years were edentulous, with large geographic variations, indicated that the oral health goals for the year 2000 suggested by the World Health Organization/Federation Dentaire International were far from being met in large areas of Norway when the data were collected (1996 to 1999) [12]. Current United States statistics from the Centers for Disease Control and Prevention (CDC) suggest that 50% of subjects aged 65 years or older have most of their teeth (ie, 23 or more) remaining [13]. However, these statistics do not include nursing home residents and are based on self-reports. The United States appears to exhibit large geographic differences in edentulousness, from approximately 10% in Hawaii to 50% in some Southern states. The CDC report anticipates that the rate of edentulousness will increase in older subjects, because many of them lack or will eventually lose dental insurance and be unable to afford dental (periodontal) care.

One of several problems with clinical periodontal research is the question of whether clinical measures of periodontitis can accurately predict the progression of disease. Any measure of dental or periodontal disease is in principle a surrogate measure aimed at assessing tooth mortality. Tooth loss may occur for many reasons and may be difficult to assess in clinical trials. For example, teeth may be lost as a consequence of (1) disease progress (ie, caries becoming endodontic lesions; periodontitis resulting in advanced bone loss, tooth mobility, and loss of function; acute inflammatory exacerbation), (2) prosthetic indications (irrational to treat), and (3) economic and social realities. With regard to the progression of periodontitis in older subjects, probing attachment loss cannot be confirmed as a valid surrogate measure for tooth loss [14]. At the same time, there appears to be an explanatory relationship between a past history of tooth loss and the extent of alveolar bone loss in older subjects [6]. Radiographic assessments might thus be more useful than clinical periodontal measures. However, rarely is the extent of alveolar bone loss defined from radiographic measurements and accounted for in epidemiologic studies.

Age-related alterations in the periodontium are not inevitably manifested as loss of probing attachment or alveolar bone [15]. In fact, data suggest that subjects who are clinically healthy from a periodontal perspective may have a continuous increase in the distance between the alveolar bone level and the cement-enamel junction (CEJ) to about the age of 50, with no additional increase in this distance thereafter [16]. Using mean values at different age groups and two standard deviations may provide upper ranges for what can be considered a normal distance between bone level and CEJ.

In older subjects, this process may be more difficult, because the response to infection may not be reflected in probing depth. In older subjects, it appears that interproximal recession and loss of attachment and alveolar bone run parallel, resulting in destruction of the periodontium in the absence of increased probing depth [16]. Longitudinal studies of older subjects (≥60 years) in Australia demonstrated that subjects with diabetes are at greater risk for attachment loss, but also that most attachment loss can be attributed to increase in gingival recession [7].

The susceptibility and severity of periodontitis are defined by three major factors: (1) the microbiologic infection, (2) host-intrinsic factors, including genetic predisposition to inflammatory responses, and (3) extrinsic factors (eg, behavioral, socioeconomic factors).

The microbiologic etiology of periodontitis in the elderly

One early experimental gingivitis study [17] showed that supragingival plaque developed faster in older subjects (65–78 years) than in young subjects (20–24 years). This finding might be explained in part by differences in periodontal status but could also suggest that growth conditions in older subjects favor rapid colonization of aerobic bacteria. The infectious etiology to chronic periodontitis in adults is well established and illustrated by a large number of reports [18–20]. Presently, the primary focus of study of infection and periodontitis is on three pathogens forming the "red complex" (*Porphyromonas gingivalis, Tannerella forsythia,* and *Treponema denticola*), which have been associated with established chronic periodontitis. It remains unclear whether the colonization pattern of these pathogens differs between younger and older adults. *T. forsythia* appears to be common both in older subjects with gingivitis only and those with periodontitis [21]. The occurrence of *P. gingivalis* has been shown to increase with age, whereas the levels of *Actinobacillus actinomycetemcomitans*, a pathogen associated with aggressive periodontitis in young adults, decrease with increasing age [22].

The immune system and periodontitis in the elderly

A decline in immune responses occurs with aging. Immune characteristic changes in older subjects are complex, encompassing an increase in serum immunoglobulin levels, a switch from naive to memory T lymphocytes, an increase in serum natural killer cells, and an increase in interleukin (IL)-1, IL-6, and tumor necrosis factor-α. Thymus-derived T lymphocytes are key cells in the adaptive immune system and are important in both the cellular and humoral immune responses to infection [23,24]. T lymphocyte levels affects mucosal responses and production of IgM antibodies and cytokines and effects a decline in phenotypic markers of T- and B-cell subsets [25]. Age-related changes in immune responses have also been reported, suggesting that peripheral blood mononuclear cell proliferation and IL-2 production decrease with age [26]. Serum IgG levels against *P. gingivalis*, a pathogen associated with periodontitis, appear to increase with age [27]. This increase may simply suggest that long-lasting exposure to the antigen is not sufficient to provide immunity against *P. gingivalis* infection. In fact, the combination of an increase in serum IgG titers and a decline in the efficacy of cellular immunity may result in an increased risk for periodontitis with increasing age. The current American Academy of Periodontology classification of periodontitis may be misleading, and there may be a need to consider specific periodontal disease patterns in the elderly subject. Pronounced gingival recession affecting interproximal spaces in combination with alveolar bone and attachment loss in older subjects may be explained by immune responses to periodontal infection that differ from those in younger adults [28].

Self-perception, quality of life, and periodontitis in the elderly

Chronic periodontitis is a slowly progressive disease. It is unclear whether cultural and historical factors affect a subject's perception of disease progression. If a subject perceives periodontitis as an unavoidable disease, this self-perception undermines any attempt at prevention. Interestingly, older subjects appear to have a rather accurate self-perception of their risks for periodontitis progression and future tooth loss [29]. Social and ethnic characteristics are major contributory and explanatory factors to the severity of periodontitis in older subjects. These findings are supported by other studies of the self-perceived benefits of periodontal health, including studies in younger subjects seeking specialist care [12].

Self-efficacy can be defined as an individual's perception of control over his or her well being and ability to perform specific forms of health behavior to effect a change in health outcomes. Major efforts must be dedicated to improving health self-perceptions and understanding of periodontal treatment needs. Tools for defining self-efficacy and means for improving health knowledge, attitudes, and behavior are cost-effective ways of reducing the impact of social factors on the prevalence and severity of periodontal disease. The response to therapy may be enhanced when clinicians consider treatment alternatives that are consistent with the limitations of the patient's self-efficacy—especially when treating older subjects.

Periodontal disease and tooth loss clearly have a significant impact on quality of life. This impact may be even more pronounced in older subjects, who may have limited financial resources and be at risk for social isolation. They may have good self-perception of their periodontal status but do not seek care because they believe it would be too expensive. The likelihood of this scenario is high, as illustrated by studies showing that older subjects without dental insurance (approximately 60% of the older United States population) may not seek regular dental care [30]. Thus, as the older dentate population increases in proportion to the total population, its access to dental care may decrease, with significant health and social consequences.

Socioeconomic status and periodontitis in the elderly

A recent analysis of the NHANES III data set, which included only those subjects who received a full periodontal examination and were older than 50 years (19.7% older than 69), demonstrated that the relationship between severity of periodontitis and socioeconomic status is modified by ethnicity. Higher-income African Americans (sic) had more periodontitis than did low-income African Americans, higher-income non-Hispanic whites, and Hispanics [31]. Hence, other reports on a direct relationship between the severity of periodontitis and socioeconomic status may be only partially correct [32].

Unfortunately, few studies have clarified the relationship between periodontal status and socioeconomic factors in older subjects while taking into account social, political, and historical factors. Such studies are urgently needed, given the increasing number of older subjects in society and their lack of dental insurance. Although Sweden has had nationwide generalized dental insurance for many years, a study from that nation demonstrated that low-income subjects have more severe periodontitis than subjects with higher income, suggesting that economic factors alone may not determine patient care or who seeks care [33]. This principle is illustrated by a study of Medicaid recipients in Kitsap County, Washington, who, responding to a questionnaire, placed dental care needs at the bottom of a priority list and stated that tooth loss was inevitable [34]. It appears that dental health care insurance or access to care alone will not resolve the disparities in oral health.

Smoking and periodontitis in the elderly

Major efforts have been dedicated to informing patients about the negative impact of smoking. Such efforts may be unsuccessful in older subjects who have an intact dentition with few, if any, signs of periodontitis. From a self-perception of risk and a self-efficacy perspective, it is difficult to convince such subjects that there are benefits to quitting smoking for periodontal reasons alone. Notwithstanding, dentists providing care for older subjects should make efforts to inform them about the benefits of stopping tobacco use.

During the past 20 years, our perception of the role of smoking in the development and progression of periodontitis has been revised. Smoking previously was not considered a key factor for periodontitis, but a large volume of studies now demonstrate that subjects who smoke cigarettes are at a higher risk for periodontitis than nonsmokers. However, studies also have shown that, although smoking has an impact on alveolar bone loss, and a dose response curve appears to exist between smoking habits and severity of periodontitis, this relationship almost disappears when one controls for current oral hygiene levels [35]. Thus, oral hygiene may have a dominating impact on the susceptibility to periodontitis, with smoking as a factor that only partially contributes to elevated risk for the disease.

Recent studies of a large group of smokers and nonsmokers demonstrate that smokers have an increased risk for bleeding on probing, in combination with poor oral hygiene [36]. Measurements of probing depth as an outcome measure for periodontitis severity in smokers and nonsmokers may therefore reflect the severity of gingivitis and pseudopocketing, rather than irreversible effects on the periodontium. Studies of the effect of nonsurgical treatment in heavy smokers and nonsmokers have shown similar effects, including reduction of probing depth [37]. The impact of smoking on periodontal conditions is difficult to assess. It has been shown that less than 10% of low-income subjects between 65 and 75 are current smokers. If current and past smokers were merged into one group, the proportion of subjects with a history of smoking in this generation might reach approximately 40% [38]. Unpublished data from the study suggest that it might take 30 years of smoking or more to have an impact on periodontal conditions; by contrast, smoking had a remarkable impact on cardiovascular status in this study group.

Systemic diseases and periodontitis in the elderly

Recent studies have suggested associations between periodontitis and systemic diseases. Specifically, diabetes mellitus, osteoporosis, and cardio-vascular diseases, including stroke, are common in older subjects. Thus, periodontitis may be a risk factor for significant systemic diseases.

Cardiovascular diseases

An association between periodontitis and cardiovascular diseases has been demonstrated in several studies [39–41]. The shared etiology may be found in a commonality of pathogens involved in periodontitis and cardiovascular disease. Thus, studies have shown that pathogens associated with periodontitis, including *P. gingivalis, Eikenella corrodens, Prevotella intermedia*, and *Streptococcus sanguis,* share the ability to invade human coronary endothelial cells [42]. Such micro-organisms may influence atherosclerotic plaque morphology, predisposing to plaque disruption and triggering an acute coronary syndrome or ischemic stroke. Furthermore, elevated serum cholesterol values have been associated with elevated serum IgG titers to *P. gingivalis* (odds ratio 7.0), suggesting that *P. gingivalis* is a factor in atherosclerosis [43].

One way in which dentists can determine whether their patients have evidence of carotid calcification as a sign of cardiovascular disease is to learn how to use panoramic radiography for the identification of this problem [44]. A significant association between radiographic signs of carotid calcification and a gold standard (duplex sonography) establishes the accuracy of this method [45]. Furthermore, studies of older subjects have shown associations between radiographic evidence of carotid calcification, a history of cardiovascular disease, and periodontitis [46].

Diabetes mellitus

The incidence of type II diabetes mellitus is increasing, perhaps as a result of changes in life-style and dietary habits leading to obesity. Recent data suggest that the prevalence of diagnosed and undiagnosed diabetes mellitus in older subjects approaches 20% [47]. Patients with diabetes mellitus are likely to develop long-term complications as a consequence of the disease. The major complications resulting from hyperglycemia include retinopathy, nephropathy, neuropathy, and circulatory abnormalities. Hyperinsulinemia in elderly type II diabetes mellitus patients has also been associated with cardiovascular disease. An elevated mortality has been reported for middle-aged patients with a combination of obesity, hypertension, and diabetes [48]. A unique cluster of metabolic abnormalities in subjects with diabetes, including dyslipidemia, hypertension, insulin resistance, and hyperglycemia, may be linked to their increased risk for other diseases, such as cardiovascular disease and chronic periodontitis [49].

Subjects with diabetes mellitus are at greater risk for destructive periodontal disease [50]. However, most studies on the relationship between periodontitis and diabetes mellitus have been performed in subjects with type I diabetes mellitus. Older subjects are predominantly at risk for type II diabetes mellitus. Few studies have reported on the relationship between periodontal disease and type II diabetes. Several of these studies reported specifically on the Pima Indians of the Gila River Indian Community in Arizona. Studies of older subjects with diabetes mellitus are limited. In a 5-year study of subjects older than 60 years, those with diabetes mellitus appeared to experience more clinical attachment loss. In this study of older subjects, smoking was not a confounding factor, supporting the aforementioned observation that older smokers may not be at greater risk for progressive periodontitis [7]. In another study of older subjects that included type II diabetes mellitus, no differences in periodontal health in relation to controls were reported [51]. The role of poor oral hygiene in subjects with diabetes mellitus might outweigh the impact of both diabetes mellitus and other factors, such as smoking [52].

Osteoporosis

Changes in alveolar bone height have been associated with systemic changes in bone tissues and osteoporosis in postmenopausal women [53]. Systemic osteopenia or osteoporosis is a degenerative disease that primarily affects postmenopausal women but also can affect older men. The disease is characterized by a loss of bone mineral density, resulting in a hip fracture. The diagnosis of osteopenia or osteoporosis is often made using bone density measurements. Approximately 20 million people in the United States have osteoporosis, with 2 million fractures each year. Several factors have been associated with osteoporosis, including female gender, age, ethnicity, diet, and life-style [54]. A diagnosis of osteoporosis is often difficult to verify, and many older people may have osteoporosis without knowing it. Subjects with a self-reported history of osteoporotic fractures also tend to have increased resorption and thinning of the mandibular lower cortex [55], and this is correlated with bone mass changes [56]. Oral osteopenia (bone loss of the jaws) may therefore be a component of systemic osteopenia and osteoporosis.

An index has been developed to assess osteoporosis using panoramic radiographs [57]. Recent studies have suggested an association between osteoporosis and periodontitis [38]. Assessment of the mandibular cortex by panoramic radiographs might be a feasible clinical method for identifying subjects who have osteopenia or osteoporosis. Paired with dental evidence of tooth loss and alveolar bone loss, such findings should justify a referral of older subjects to a clinic for further evaluation of osteoporosis.

Risk profile

The susceptibility to periodontitis and to other systemic diseases varies with a large number of factors. It has been suggested that genetic factors explain 50% of cases of periodontitis. Although it might be possible to assess genetic factors in younger subjects by studying periodontitis severity in their parents, it would, of course, be difficult to obtain valid information about periodontitis in the parents of currently old patients. The risk for periodontitis and the impact of disease susceptibility in currently older subjects are obvious, whereas future periodontitis risk may depend on other factors than those applying to younger patients. Therefore, dentists should develop skills to identify older subjects who may be at risk for an unsuccessful aging process.

This review of factors associated with periodontitis makes it clear that a periodontal risk profile for older subjects can be established:

Poor oral hygiene remains a significant determinant independent of age.
Low socioeconomic status is an important factor.
Older African Americans are more likely to have an elevated risk for periodontitis than other ethnic groups.
Older men appear to be at greater risk than older women.
In combination with poor oral hygiene, a smoking habit is probably detrimental.
Older subjects with a history of cardiovascular disease, diabetes mellitus, or osteoporosis probably have an elevated risk.
Subjects with negative self-perception and self-efficacy are at greater risk.

Dentists can only have an impact on three of these factors: poor oral hygiene, smoking habits, and systemic conditions. It therefore seems reasonable to direct the major efforts to reduce the risks of periodontitis toward improvement of oral hygiene, while also working with older patients on smoking cessation. Dentists can improve older patients' self-perception of oral health and self-efficacy by providing information and support. Referral of older patients with established periodontitis and risk profiles for systemic diseases should be a routine procedure for dentists. Coordinated medical and dental care would increase the quality of life for such older patients. Such coordinated treatment plans may require that dentists consider alternative options for dental treatment. Dental care should probably be focused on control of the oral infectious burden as a primary goal and reconstruction as a secondary one. Improvement of periodontal status improves quality of life [58].

Summary

The increasing population of older subjects with dental care needs will become a major challenge to our society and its care providers. To manage the health care needs of the elderly, a coordination between medical and dental care providers will become necessary. From the dental perspective, it is important to develop skills in the risk assessment of older patients. Such risk assessment of older subjects should take an approach that is holistic and focused on the reduction of the infectious burden and the improvement of self-efficacy.

References

[1] Reinhardt UE, Hussey PS, Anderson GF. US health care spending in an international context. Health Aff 2004;23(3):10–25.

[2] The Surgeon General's Report on Oral Health in America. Available at: http://www.nidcr.nih.gov/NewsandReports/NewsRelease052000.htm. Accessed January 24, 2005.

[3] Available at: http://www.cms.hhs.gov/statistics/nhe/historical/highlights.asp.

[4] Armitage GC. Periodontal diagnoses and classification of periodontal disease. Periodontology 2000 2004;34(1):1–9.

[5] Renvert S, Persson GR. A systematic review of the use of residual probing depth, bleeding on probing and furcation status following initial periodontal therapy to predict further attachment and tooth loss. J Clin Periodontol 2002;29(Suppl 3):82–9.

[6] Persson GR, Persson RE, MacEntee CI, et al. Periodontitis and perceived risk for periodontitis in older subjects with evidence of depression. J Clin Periodontol 2003;30:691–6.

[7] Thomson WM, Slade GD, Beck JD, et al. Incidence of periodontal attachment loss over 5 years among older South Australians. J Clin Periodontol 2004;31:119–25.

[8] Albandar JM, Brunelle JA, Kingman A. Destructive periodontal disease in adults 30 years of age and older in the United States, 1988–1994. J Periodontol 1999;70:13–29.

[9] Hirotomo T, Yoshihara A, Yano M, et al. Longitudinal study on periodontal conditions in healthy elderly people in Japan. Community Dent Oral Epidemiol 2002;30:409–17.

[10] Mack F, Mojon P, Budz-Jörgensen E, et al. Caries and periodontal disease of the elderly in Pomerania, Germany: results of the Study of Health in Pomerania. Gerodontology 2004;21:27–36.

[11] Takata Y, Ansai T, Awano S, et al. Relationship of physical fitness to chewing in an 80-year-old population. Oral Dis 2004;10:44–9.

[12] Henriksen BM, Axell T, Laake K. Geographic differences in tooth loss and denture-wearing among the elderly in Norway. Community Dent Oral Epidemiol 2003;31:403–11.

[13] Anonymous. Centers for Medicare and Medicaid Services. US Department of Health and Human Services. Available at: www.cms.hhs.gov/statistics/nhe/. Accessed January 24, 2005.

[14] Hujoel PP, Leroux BG, DeRouen TA, et al. Evaluating the validity of probing attachment loss as a surrogate for tooth mortality in a clinical trial on the elderly. J Dent Res 1997;76:858–66.

[15] Papapanou PN, Lindhe J, Sterrett JD, et al. Considerations on the contribution of aging to loss of periodontal tissue support. J Clin Periodontol 1991;18:611–5.

[16] Persson RE, Hollender LG, Persson GR. Assessment of alveolar bone levels from intraoral radiographs in subjects between ages 15 and 94 years seeking dental care. J Clin Periodontol 1998;25:647–54.

[17] Holm-Pedersen P, Agerbaek N, Theilade E. Experimental gingivitis in young and elderly individuals. J Clin Periodontol 1975;2:14–24.

[18] Haffajee AD, Cugini MA, Tanner A, et al. Subgingival microbiota in healthy, well-maintained elder and periodontitis subjects. J Clin Periodontol 1998;25:346–53.

[19] Socransky SS, Haffajee AD. Evidence of bacterial etiology: a historical perspective. Periodontology 2000 1994;5:7–25.

[20] Socransky SS, Haffajee AD. Dental biofilms: difficult therapeutic targets. Periodontology 2000 2002;28:12–55.

[21] Persson GR, Schlegel-Bregenzer B, Chung WO, et al. Serum antibody titers to *Bacteroides forsythus* in elderly subjects with gingivitis or periodontitis. J Clin Periodontol 2000;27:839–45.

[22] Rodenburg JP, van Winkelhoff AJ, Winkel EG, et al. Occurrence of *Bacteroides gingivalis*, *Bacteroides intermedius*, and *Actinobacillus actinomycetemcomitans* in severe periodontitis in relation to age and treatment history. J Clin Periodontol 1990;17:351–5.

[23] Huber LA, Xu QB, Jurgens G, et al. Correlation of lymphocyte lipid composition membrane microviscosity and mitogen response in the aged. Eur J Immunol 1991;21:2761–5.

[24] McArthur WP, Bloom K, Taylor M, et al. Peripheral blood leukocyte populations in the elderly with and without periodontal disease. J Clin Periodontol 1996;23:846–52.

[25] Percival RS, Marsh PD, Challacombe SJ. Serum antibodies to commensal oral and gut bacteria vary with age. FEMS Immunol Med Microbiol 1996;15:35–42.

[26] Beharka AA, Paiva S, Leka LS, et al. Effect of age on the gastrointestinal-associated mucosal immune response of humans. J Gerontol A Biol Sci Med Sci 2001;56:B218–23.

[27] De Nardin AM, Sojar HT, Grossi SG, et al. Humoral immunity of older adults with periodontal disease to Porphyromonas gingivalis. Infect Immun 1991;59:4363–70.

[28] Schlegel-Bregenzer B, Persson RE, Persson GR. Gingivitis and periodontitis in elderly subjects. Clinical and microbiological findings. J Clin Periodontol 1998;25:895–907.

[29] Kiyak HA, Persson RE, Persson GR. Influences on the perceptions of and responses to periodontal disease among older adults. Periodontology 1998;16:34–43.

[30] Manski RJ, Goodman HS, Reid BC, et al. Dental insurance visits and expenditures among older adults. Am J Public Health 2004;94:759–64.

[31] Borrell LN, Burt BA, Neigbors HW, et al. Social factors and periodontitis in an older population. Am J Public Health 2004;94:748–54.

[32] Genco RJ, Ho AW, Grossi SG, et al. Relationship of stress, distress and inadequate coping behaviors to periodontal disease. J Periodontol 1999;70:711–23.

[33] Norderyd O, Hugoson A, Grusovin G. Risk of severe periodontal disease in a Swedish adult population. A longitudinal study. J Clin Periodontol 1999;26:608–15.

[34] Hansson W, Persson GR. Periodontal conditions and service utilization behaviors in a low income population. Oral Health Prev Dent 2003;1:99–109.

[35] Bolin A, Eklund G, Frithiof L, et al. The effect of changed smoking habits on marginal alveolar bone loss. A longitudinal study. Swed Dent J 1993;17:211–6.

[36] Amarasena N, Ekanayaka AN, Herath L, et al. Association between smoking, betel chewing and gingival bleeding in rural Sri Lanka. J Clin Periodontol 2003;30:403–8.

[37] Preber H, Bergström J. Effect of non-surgical treatment on gingival bleeding in smokers and non-smokers. Acta Odontol Scand 1986;44:85–9.

[38] Persson RE, Hollender LG, Powell LV, et al. Assessment of periodontal and systemic health comparing panoramic radiography and self-reported history in older persons. I. Focus on osteoporosis. J Clin Periodontol 2002;29:796–802.

[39] DeStefano F, Anda RF, Kahn HS, et al. Dental disease and risk of coronary heart disease and mortality. Br Med J 1993;306:688–91.

[40] Mattila KJ. Dental infections as a risk factor for acute myocardial infarction. Eur Heart J 1993;14(Suppl K):51–3.

[41] Beck J, Garcia R, Heiss G, et al. Periodontal disease and cardiovascular disease. J Periodontol 1996;67:1123–37.

[42] Dorn BR, Dunn WA Jr, Progulske-Fox A. Invasion of human coronary artery cells by periodontal pathogens. Infect Immun 1999;67:5792–8.

[43] Cutler CW, Shinedling EA, Nunn M, et al. Association between periodontitis and hyperlipidemia: cause or effect? J Periodontol 1999;70:1429–34.

[44] Cohen SN, Friedlander AH, Jolly DA, et al. Carotid calcification on panoramic radiographs: an important marker for vascular risk. Oral Surg Oral Med Oral Pathol Oral Radiol Endod 2002;94:510–4.

[45] Ravon N, Hollender LG, Persson GR. Signs of carotid calcification from dental panoramic radiography are in agreement with Doppler sonography results. J Clin Periodontol 2003;29: 1084–90.

[46] Persson RE, Hollender LG, Powell LV, et al. Assessment of periodontal and systemic health comparing panoramic radiographs and self-reported history in older persons. II. Focus on cardiovascular diseases. J Clin Periodontol 2002;29:803–10.

[47] Resnick HE, Shorr RI, Kuller L, et al. Prevalence and clinical implications of American Diabetes Association–defined diabetes and other categories of glucose dysregulation in older adults: the health, aging and body composition study. J Clin Epidemiol 2001;54:869–76.

[48] Aldridge NB, Stump TE, Nothwehr FK, et al. Prevalence and outcomes of comorbid metabolic and cardiovascular conditions in middle- and older-age adults. J Clin Epidemiol 2001;54:928–34.

[49] Kendall DM, Bergenstal RM. Comprehensive management of patients with type 2 diabetes: establishing priorities of care. Am J Manag Care 2001;7(Suppl 10):S327–43.

[50] Taylor GW, Burt BA, Becker MP, et al. Severe periodontitis and risk for poor glycemic control in patients with non–insulin-dependent diabetes mellitus. J Periodontol 1996;67: 1085–93.

[51] Persson RE, Hollender LG, MacEntee MI, et al. Assessment of periodontal and systemic health comparing panoramic radiographs and self-reported history in older persons. Focus on diabetes mellitus. J Clin Periodontol 2003;30:207–13.

[52] Karikoski A, Ilanne-Parikka P, Murtomaa H. Oral self-care and periodontal health indicators among adults with diabetes in Finland. Acta Odontol Scand 2001;59:390–5.

[53] Pilgram TK, Hildebolt CF, Yokoyama-Crothers N, et al. Relationships between longitudinal changes in radiographic alveolar bone height and probing depth measurements: data from postmenopausal women. J Periodontol 1999;70:829–33.

[54] Smeets-Goevaers CG, Lesusink GL, Papapoulos SE, et al. The prevalence of low bone mineral density in Dutch perimenopausal women: the Eindhoven perimenopausal osteoporosis study. Osteoporos Int 1998;8:404–9.

[55] Bollen AM, Taguchi A, Hujoel PP, et al. Case-control study on self-reported osteoporotic fractures and mandibular cortical bone. Oral Surg Oral Med Oral Pathol Oral Radiol Endod 2000;90:518–24.

[56] Civitelli R, Pilgram TK, Dotson M, et al. Alveolar and postcranial bone density in postmenopausal women receiving hormone/estrogen replacement therapy: a randomized, double-blind, placebo-controlled trial. Arch Intern Med 2002;162:1409–15.

[57] Klemetti E, Kolmakov S, Kroger H. Pantomography in assessment of the osteoporosis risk group. Scand J Dent Res 1994;102:68–72.

[58] Needleman I, McGrath G, Floyd P, et al. Impact of oral health on the life quality of periodontal patients. J Clin Periodontol 2004;31:454–7.

ELSEVIER
SAUNDERS

THE DENTAL
CLINICS
OF NORTH AMERICA

Dent Clin N Am 49 (2005) 293–308

Dental Caries in Older Adults

Ralph H. Saunders, Jr, DDS, MS[a,b,*],
Cyril Meyerowitz, BDS, MS[a,c]

[a]*Eastman Department of Dentistry, University of Rochester,
625 Elmwood Avenue, Rochester, NY 14620, USA*
[b]*Monroe Community Hospital, 435 East Henrietta Road, Rochester, NY 14620, USA*
[c]*Eastman Dental Center, 625 Elmwood Avenue, Rochester, NY 14620, USA*

Dental caries has become a significant oral health problem for older adults. This development is due in part to the increasing longevity of the population and the increases in tooth retention in this age group. In 1962, 60% of the community-based population of the United States over age 65 was edentulous [1]. By 1985, the proportion had declined to 42% [2]. The National Health and Nutrition Examination Study (NHANES) III survey of 1988 to 1991 found that only 26.0% (±3.0%) of subjects aged 65 to 69 and 31.1% (3.0%) of those aged 70 to 74 [3] were edentulous. This increase in the number of teeth increases the number of surfaces at risk for caries development.

This article reviews the causes, prevalence, and incidence of both coronal and root surface caries, identifies risk factors, and discusses new approaches to prevention and treatment of caries in older adults.

Etiology

Dental caries, which can affect both the root and the coronal part of the tooth, is clinically defined as a lesion that extends beyond the surface of enamel or cementum and is identified by being penetrable with the dental explorer and by discoloration ranging from white to deep brown. Caries in some locations (eg, interproximal) also can be identified as an area of increased lucency on a dental radiograph or digital image.

The mechanism of development of coronal and root caries in older adults appears to be similar to that in younger populations. It starts with

---

* Corresponding author. Eastman Department of Dentistry, University of Rochester, 625 Elmwood Avenue, Rochester, NY 14620.
  E-mail address: ralph_saunders@urmc.rochester.edu (R.H. Saunders).

demineralization of enamel or cementum by organic acids (eg, lactic, acetic), which are produced over time when bacteria in plaque metabolize fermentable carbohydrates. The lesion can be remineralized and arrested, or it can progress into dentin [4]. However, the development of caries in older adults differs from that in younger individuals in that the elderly have numerous additional risk factors (see further discussion) that increase their susceptibility to caries.

Prevalence and incidence

Coronal caries (prevalence)

The prevalence of dental caries is its frequency in a population. Establishing the prevalence is important for assessing the treatment need at a particular point in time. The most recent comprehensive and representative examination of the prevalence of oral health conditions in the United States community-based adult population was the NHANES III of 1988 to 1991 [3]. In this study, 14,604 community-based individuals aged 18 years and older were surveyed. Table 1 presents the number of carious coronal surfaces by age group for the total population and by ethnic group as established by the NHANES III study.

Compared with an earlier survey by the National Institute for Dental Research (NIDR) [2], which presented results by different age groups, levels of coronal caries appeared to be higher in the NHANES study. The difference may relate to better general health among the employed adults in the earlier survey. As noted in the NHANES report, comparing these findings for caries with those in other surveys is problematic because of differences in the racial and ethnic composition of survey populations, in oral health summary measures, and in whether the index was applied to the total sample or limited to the dentate sample. However, it is clear that older minorities in the United States population have disproportionately more

Table 1
Coronal caries by age group

Age group (y)	Total population Number (SD) of decayed surfaces	Non-Hispanic white Number (SD) of decayed surfaces	Non-Hispanic black Number (SD) of decayed surfaces	Mexican American Number (SD) of decayed surfaces
18–24	1.6 (0.2)	1.4 (0.2)	2.4 (0.2)	1.9 (0.2)
25–34	2.1 (0.1)	1.8 (0.2)	3.5 (0.4)	2.1 (0.2)
35–44	1.9 (0.2)	1.7 (0.3)	3.5 (0.4)	2.6 (0.3)
45–54	1.6 (0.6)	1.4 (0.2)	2.9 (0.6)	3.1 (0.5)
55–64	1.6 (0.2)	1.2 (0.2)	4.1 (1.0)	4.1 (0.4)
65–74	1.6 (0.3)	1.2 (0.2)	3.8 (0.9)	3.8 (0.6)
75+	1.7 (0.2)	1.5 (0.2)	4.3 (1.0)	3.5 (0.8)

Abbreviation: SD, standard deviation.

From Ezzati T, Massey J, Waxsberg J, et al. Sample design: Third National Health and Nutrition Examination Survey. Vital Health Stat 2 1992;1(32); with permission.

coronal caries than whites. The reasons for the differences by race and ethnicity were not explored in this study but may partially reflect differences in the availability of oral health services.

Root surface caries (prevalence)

Root surface caries is more prevalent among older adults than any other age group. The presence of gingival recession, epidemic in this age group, and other risk factors (to be discussed later) leads to the very high susceptibility of the elderly. The prevalence of root surface caries in the NHANES report is displayed in Table 2.

The levels of root caries noted here are similar to those in the 1985 NIDR study. As with coronal caries, non-Hispanic whites have the lowest number of untreated root caries surfaces.

Caries prevalence in nursing home elderly

At any one time, approximately 5% of people aged 65 and over in the United States reside in nursing homes. However, it is estimated that 43% of this age group will have a nursing home admission during their lifetime.

Most surveys indicate that the elderly who reside in nursing homes or other institutions have the worst oral health of any subpopulation in this age group. Table 3 displays the prevalence of caries in several recent surveys and confirms high levels of caries in this population [5–9].

Caries incidence

Caries incidence refers to the development of new lesions over time. The rate of development of new caries in coronal and root surfaces is higher in older adults than in younger populations [10].

Table 2
Root surface caries by age group

Age group (y)	Total Number (SD) of decayed surfaces	Non-Hispanic whites Number (SD) of decayed surfaces	Non-Hispanic blacks Number (SD) of decayed surfaces	Mexican Americans Number (SD) of decayed surfaces
18–24	0.3 (0.1)	0.3 (0.1)	0.5 (0.1)	0.4 (0.1)
25–34	0.5 (0.1)	0.5 (0.1)	1.1 (0.2)	0.5 (0.1)
35–44	0.7 (0.1)	0.7 (0.1)	1.3 (0.3)	0.9 (0.2)
45–54	0.8 (0.1)	0.6 (0.1)	1.3 (0.3)	1.5 (0.4)
55–64	1.0 (0.2)	0.8 (0.2)	2.3 (0.7)	2.6 (0.6)
64–75	0.9 (0.1)	0.6 (0.1)	2.5 (0.6)	2.4 (0.5)
75+	1.5 (0.2)	1.3 (0.2)	4.1 (1.6)	1.7 (0.6)

Abbreviation: SD, standard deviation.
From Ezzati T, Massey J, Waxsberg J, et al. Sample design: Third National Health and Nutrition Examination Survey. Vital Health Stat 2 1992;1(32); with permission.

Table 3
Dental caries in recent nursing home surveys

Survey	N	Site	Prevalence
Chalmers et al 2002 [5]	224	Adelaide	Mean no. decayed surfaces/dentate subject: Coronal 1.7 Root 1.5
Wyatt et al 2002 [6]	369	Vancouver	50.4% with coronal caries 68.8% with root caries
Saub et al 2001 [7]	175	Melbourne	46% with coronal caries 30% with root caries
Frankl et al 2000 [8]	412	Avon	63% with root caries
Weyant et al 1993 [9]	650	United States	Percentage of dentate with decayed or filled sufaces: Coronal 93.0% Root 56.2%

Table 4 displays the results of several surveys [10–17]. Comparison among them is hampered by their use of different units of caries measurement. Nonetheless, the high incidence of coronal and root caries is evident. Similarly, a meta-analysis of four surveys of older adults observed that the combined incidence of coronal and root caries was greater than that in recent cohort studies of adolescents [10].

In summary, surveys demonstrate that the prevalence of coronal caries is as high in the elderly as in other groups of adults, whereas the prevalence of root surface caries is much higher. Whites in the United States have significantly lower levels of both coronal and root caries than do Hispanics and African Americans. Studies of incidence illustrate a greater ongoing development of both types of lesion in the elderly than in other populations. Finally, older residents of nursing homes have more coronal and root caries than those who reside in the community.

Significance of caries to health and economics

It would be difficult to overstate the significance that caries now has in the elderly because of increases in longevity and tooth retention. Caries has been identified as the major cause of tooth loss in older adults [18]. Tooth loss, in turn, is the most significant negative variable in oral health–related quality of life for the elderly [19].

The presence of caries in the elderly has also been associated with several general health conditions. For instance, a 5-year longitudinal survey of 528 community-dwelling adults aged 60 years or more residing in South Australia revealed that chronic use of anti-asthma and beta-blocking medications was related to an increase in coronal caries. Root caries was not affected [13].

Table 4
Coronal and root caries incidence in older adults

Study	N	Location	Period	Coronal caries	Root caries
Thomson 2004 [10]	Meta-analysis	...	3 y	0.5 – 0.8 surfaces affected/year	0.2 – 0.4 surfaces affected/year
Fure 2003 [11]	102	Sweden	10 y	Decrease w/age	Increase w/age
Chalmers et al 2002 [12]	215	Australia	1 y	3.5 DS dementia 1.4 DS no dementia	1.7 DS dementia 0.8 DS no dementia
Thomson 2002 [13]	528	New Zealand	5 y	2.2 DS	1.9 DS
Luan et al 2000 [14]	440	China	10 y	66%–96% with 1+ new lesions	
Drake et al 1997 [15]	452	North Carolina	3 y	Blacks: 0.8 S/100 SAR White: 1.6 S/100 SAR	...
Lawrence et al 1996 [16]	702	North Carolina	5 y	...	39% of blacks affected 52% of whites affected
Hand et al 1988 [17]	451	Iowa	1.5 y	1.4 S/100 SAR	2.6 S/100 SAR

Abbreviations: DS, decayed surfaces; S/100 SAR, surfaces affected per 100 surfaces at risk.

In a comparison between 24 Michigan adults with Type II+ diabetes and 18 healthy adults, the latter tended to have less caries; those with well-controlled diabetes had a tendency toward less caries than those who were poorly controlled. None of the differences, however, were statistically significant [20]. Serum albumin levels have been recognized as a screening measure for general health and mortality. In a study of 763 randomly selected older adults in Japan, serum albumin was compared with the prevalence of coronal and root surface caries among the subjects. Results showed an inverse correlation of root caries prevalence with serum albumin level adjusted for age, basal metabolism index, and concentration of IgG [21]. Maupome et al [22] compared the presence of immunologic disease, osteoporosis, arthritis, cerebrovascular attack (CVA), hypertension, and cardiovascular disease to caries prevalence. The investigators found a statistically significant association between caries (no discrimination between coronal and root surface) and CVA, but not between caries and the other conditions. Dental caries has marked economic significance for older adults, because oral infections, including caries and their sequelae, account for the major portion of their annual dental expenditures [23].

Current evidence indicates that both coronal and root surface caries are significant for older adults because they are the primary causes of tooth loss. Although some relationships between caries and general health exist, additional research is needed better to characterize the associations and relationships. Caries is particularly significant in the elderly because it accounts for most of the oral health expenditures of this population, which pays most dental fees out of pocket.

Risk factors

Older adults have considerably more factors that place tooth surfaces at risk for caries than do younger adults, because of the many conditions faced by this population during the last phase of life, which can last as long as 40 years. During that period, the elderly face a wide spectrum of oral and general health problems.

Individual conditions that are proven risk factors are listed in Table 5 [12,13,22,24–32]. Combinations of these factors, which are common in older adults, elevate the risk of caries development.

The value of recognizing risk factors was noted in a 2002 Consensus Conference that recommended management of caries by identifying the number and nature of risks and classifying patients into risk categories of high, moderate, and low [33]. Another conference recommended a separate, unique assessment in special patients for whom the risks are more variable [34]. An example of the special circumstances faced by older adults is that those who are institutionalized are offered a mean of eight sugar intakes per day [29].

Table 5
Demonstrated caries risk factors in older adults

Risk factor	Study
Attachment loss	Gilbert et al 2001 [24]
Mouth dryness	Saunders et al 1990 [25]
Presence of restorations	Morse et al 2002 [26], Gilbert et al 2001 [24]
Removable partial dentures	Jepson et al 2001 [27]
Cognitive decline	Avlund et al 2004 [28], Chalmers et al 2002 [12]
Institutionalization	Maupome et al 2003 [22], Steele et al 1998 [29]
Medical problems (stroke)	Maupome et al 2003 [22]
Geography (residents in rural setting)	Shah and Sundarum 2004 [30], Vargas et al 2003 [31]
Medications (antiasthma)	Thomson et al 2004 [13]
Literacy (low levels)	Shah and Sundarum 2004 [30]
Lack of manual dexterity	Kurzon and Preston 2004 [32]
Difficulty comprehending oral care instructions	Kurzon and Preston 2004 [32]

Although efforts to categorize patients by risk assessment are valuable, Kurzon and Preston [32] point out the difficulty of being accurate in this type of organization owing to the multiplicity of factors involved. They note that the easiest group to classify by risk assessment is patients who have marked mouth dryness. These patients are found with consistency in the highest risk category. It is important for the clinician to recognize risk factors when planning treatment for these patients.

Prevention

Prevention is as important for the control of dental caries in older adults as it is in children and adolescents. The latter groups have been studied more extensively, but the results of these studies can be extrapolated to older populations. Because coronal caries and root caries share similar or identical causative factors, preventive efforts can be directed in the same way toward both [35]. Therefore, preventive efforts can be discussed for both diseases simultaneously.

At this time, clinical decisions about prevention for older adults should be based on evidence-based research where it exists. However, given the scarcity of studies in this population, dentists also need to rely on contemporary consensus about care for these special patients. An overview of the use of preventive agents in older populations follows.

Fluoride dentifrice

Dentifrice containing approximately 1000 ppm fluoride (F) is probably the most widely used personal topical F-containing product. Its value is primarily based on the capacity of F to facilitate remineralization of tooth structure following the multiple daily challenges from acids produced by *Streptococcus mutans* and other normal oral flora.

A randomized controlled trial (RCT) involving 810 adults aged 54 years or more reported that a dentifrice containing 1100 ppm F reduced coronal caries by 41% and root caries by 67% when compared with a nonfluoride dentifrice [36].

The effectiveness of F dentifrices is influenced by a number of factors, including frequency of application, F concentration, and rinsing protocols [37]. Brushing teeth twice per day with an F-containing dentifrice appears to be the most effective method, as reported in observational studies [38] and by a 2002 consensus conference on the oral care of persons with special needs [34]. A study of F dose response has demonstrated that, for each increase in concentration of 500 ppm F in dentifrice, there is generally a further 6% to 7% reduction in caries [39]. A recent RCT demonstrated that 57% of adults with one or more root caries lesions who used a dentifrice containing 5000 ppm F for 6 months had reversal of root caries. Only 29% of those who used a dentifrice containing 1100 ppm experienced root caries reversals [40]. Rinsing the mouth after use of dentifrice is recommended, primarily to remove the particles of abrasive that are included to aid plaque removal. Rinsing should use a low volume of water, because high volumes will decrease the retention of F [41].

Fluoride rinses

Clinical trials have demonstrated that 0.5% sodium fluoride (NaF) mouth rinses can reduce both coronal and root caries in adults living in fluoridated and nonfluoridated areas [42–44].

Commercial 0.5% NaF rinses are readily available without a prescription at modest cost. They are useful to older adults with disabilities because, in addition to their function as a rinse, they can be applied using intraoral applicators [45] and, unlike dentifrices, do not require a post-use rinse with water. The NaF rinses also may have special value for this population because it is the most likely to suffer from conditions that limit saliva flow and thus enhance the retention of F [46].

Fluoride gels

Gels are colloidal agents in which an active solute (eg, F) can be suspended in a jelly-like matrix. The potential value of gels containing F or other protective caries control ingredients lies in their capacity to maintain contact with tooth surfaces for extended periods of time. Formulations commonly used are neutral NaF 5000 ppm and acidulated phosphorylated F 12,000 ppm. The efficacy of professionally applied gels has been demonstrated for management of root caries in older adults [43,44]. However, with the recently increased availability of high-concentration

(5000 ppm) dentifrices and the comparative ease of use of other agents, use of gels by this population may decline.

Fluoride varnishes

A varnish is a liquid preparation that can be applied to a solid surface and form a hard, usually transparent coating. Varnishes containing up to 22,600 ppm F are newer to preventive regimens than rinses and gels, but they have properties that encourage their use among older adults. Compared with gels, varnishes are faster and easier to apply. The therapeutic frequency of their application is reduced, their potential ingestion is easier to control, their patient acceptance is higher, and no professional prophylaxis is needed before their application [47,48]. Weintraub [49] recommends their use in special-needs patients for precisely these reasons.

When F varnish was applied once every 3 months as part of a maintenance program for adults following periodontal surgery, significantly less root caries was observed in the varnish recipients compared with controls [50]. Although they can be used as sole agents, F varnishes have shown even greater therapeutic effect in older and special needs patients when used in combination with other preventive ingredients, including chlorhexidine (CHX) varnish [51,52], CHX rinse, and CHX gel [53,54].

Other fluoride delivery systems

In addition to the systems already discussed, efforts have been undertaken to deliver F by other means, including impregnation in toothpicks and floss [55]. Mechanisms such as these require greater overall effort and dexterity and so are unlikely to become widely used by older adults.

Chlorhexidine

CHX is an antibacterial agent that is active against gram-positive and gram-negative organisms, facultative anaerobes, and yeast. In dentistry, it was used initially to control periodontal infection but was later found to be effective against cariogenic bacteria. CHX is now being used for effective caries control as a sole agent in the form of a 0.2% rinse, a 1% to 10% gel, and a 1% to 10% varnish and in combination with F in these same forms. Formulations that have been demonstrated to be especially effective with older adults include the varnish and CHX gel for control of secondary caries [56] and a combination of an F varnish with the CHX gel for control of root surface caries in institutionalized elderly [52].

Xylitol

Xylitol is a sugar with a flavor that emulates sucrose [57]. It has been shown, however, to create an unfavorable metabolic environment for

S mutans [58] and may interfere with its adherence to teeth [59]. These properties make it a good potential caries preventive agent.

Simons et al [60] found that use of a CHX/xylitol chewing gum improved plaque scores in a nursing home population. The xylitol gum alone decreased the *S mutans* count in saliva better than CHX rinse in an adult population [61]. In rats, a dentifrice with 10% xylitol combined with 1000 ppm NaF produced more dentin remineralization than F alone [62]. Xylitol is relatively new as an anticaries agent, and its use is not considered routine at this time. However, its capacity to be incorporated in gum may be of increasing interest to older adults who can safely manage chewing gum.

In summary, evidence is increasing that caries-preventive agents containing F are effective for older adults, as they have been for younger populations. With additional testing and familiarity, new products containing CHX and xylitol may come into routine use. It is important to note that the ultimate strategy for prevention of root surface caries is prevention of loss of periodontal attachment [31]. Hence, maintaining excellent periodontal health, which can minimize the number of root surfaces at risk, also is beneficial to caries prevention.

Management

Management of caries in older adults poses special challenges.

Coronal caries

Criteria for the selection of technique and materials for restoration of coronal caries in older adults are similar to those for younger populations and include size and configuration of the lesion, overall health and functional ability of the patient, caries history, expense, and aesthetic imperatives.

Characterization of lesion size and location can use Black's classification. Choices for materials include amalgam and composites for conservative lesions and crowns when half or more of the functional structure of the tooth has been lost. Often, older patients require less local anesthesia for excavation of coronal lesions than do younger patients, because of decreased size of the pulp chamber and decreased innervation; decisions on this matter must be individualized and mutual between patient and dentist. The anatomy placed and restorations may be less detailed, because of tooth wear that is physiologic with age.

Root caries

Billings et al [46] demonstrated a reliable classification of carious lesions of the root by depth toward the pulp. Using this system, they delineated four grades of depth, from 1 (superficial and not penetrable with the explorer) to 4 (entering pulp chamber) and accompanied them with appropriate management recommendations, which are summarized in Table 6.

Table 6
Management of root surface caries

	Grade I	Grade II	Grade III	Grade IV
Description	White or light brown; surface cannot be penetrated.	Light brown; 0.5 to 1.0 mm penetration.	Dark brown; penetration equal to or greater than 1 mm but not extending to pulp.	Brown or black; penetration into dental pulp.
Management	Topical fluoride and remineralizing agents; frequent recalls	Excavation of lesion, reshaping of margins, and application of topical fluoride	Restoration with glass-ionomer cement or composite resin	Endodontics or extraction

Data from Billings R, Brown L, Kaster A. Contemporary treatment strategies for root surface dental caries. Gerodontics 1985;1:20–7.

Wyatt and MacIntee [63] recommended a more subjective "extent of structural damage" classification with three levels, from low to high (Table 7).

The newest generation of dental composites and glass ionomers has significantly improved the outcomes of restorative procedures. A summary list of materials and selected properties appears in Table 8.

As mentioned previously, numerous, complex nondental risk factors apply more frequently to older adults and must be considered in caries management decisions. These include diet frequency and content, saliva flow rate, levels of *S mutans* and *lactobacilli* [64], access to preventive agents, such as frequent low-dose F [65] or CHX [66], patient education [65], and frequent recalls [65].

New and alternative caries management strategies

In addition to the preventive and restorative agents already noted, which have gained wide acceptance, new materials have emerged that may prove even more effective in the future.

For example, Holmes [67] has demonstrated the reversal of leathery root caries (noncavitated sites) in 89 subjects aged 60 to 92 years with exposure to

Table 7
Management of root caries

Extent of damage	Management
Low	Remineralization
Moderate	Restoration
High	Endodontics or extraction

Data from Wyatt C, MacEntee M. Dental caries in chronically disabled elders. Spec Care Dentist 1997;17:196–202.

Table 8
Current materials for root caries restorations for older adults

Material	Properties
Glass ionomer	Adhesive to dentin, releases fluoride
Resin-modified glass ionomer	Light cured, good early strength, easy placement
Composite resin	Best aesthetics, no fluoride release
Compomer	Single component, light curable, less fluoride release

From Burgess J, Gallo J. Treating root–surface caries. Dent Clin North Am 2002;46: 385–404; with permission.

ozone. Johnson and Almqvist [51] demonstrated that regular professional oral hygiene with F-containing prophy paste, with or without supplemental F or CHX, can prevent further progression of superficial root caries lesions and obviate the placement of restorations. A new agent, Carisolv (Medi Team AB, Skokie, Illinois), has shown potential as a solvent for carious tooth structure, both alone [68] and in combination with air-abrasion [69]. Use of Carisolv may reduce the need for rotary excavation and the attendant trauma, making restorative procedures less traumatic for older adults who already suffer from uncomfortable conditions. Another potentially less traumatic approach is atraumatic restorative treatment (ART), which uses only hand instruments for excavation, followed by restoration with glass ionomer cements. This form of provisional care, used for medically or physically compromised older adults, can make management of caries more accessible to these special older patients [70]. Hu et al [71] have recently shown that the "more viscous" glass ionomer cements used in high-risk patients can inhibit the formation of recurrent lesions for up to 24 months, even if the restoration itself has been lost. Finally, although considerable technique refinement is needed, the use of lasers for easier excavation and tooth preparation is still under evaluation [72].

Future directions

Judging from the evidence presented here, dental caries will be a significant problem for both community-based and institutionalized older adults for the foreseeable future. Improvements in prevention should come with careful testing of suggested protocols based on risk assessment.

Management of caries may be revolutionized by advances in molecular biology and genetics. The genome for *S mutans* has been elucidated [73], opening the way for modifications that may reduce its virulence. For example, a gene known as *fabM* has been found to be capable of changing its membrane composition to allow it to be more resistant to the acids it produces [74]. The possibility may soon exist of modifying *fabM* to inhibit this mechanism and render *mutans* less cariogenic.

Although they are still at the preliminary stage, such innovative approaches may be particularly useful in older patients, considering the difficulty of reducing the multiple caries risk factors in this population.

References

[1] Decayed, missing and filled teeth among persons 1–74 years. United States. NCHS Series II, No. 223, Hyattsville (MD): U.S. Department of Health and Human Services; 1981.

[2] Miller A, Brunelle J, Carlos J, et al. Oral health of United States adults: national survey of oral health in US employed adults and seniors 1985–1986. NIH Publication #87–2868. Bethesda (MD): National Institute of Health; 1987.

[3] Ezzati T, Massey J, Waxsberg J, et al. Sample design: Third National Health and Nutrition Examination Survey. Vital Health Stat 2 1992;1(32).

[4] Featherstone J. Fluoride, remineralization and root caries. Am Dent J 1994;6:271–4.

[5] Chalmers J, Hodge C, Suss J, et al. The prevalence and experience of oral diseases in Adelaide nursing home residents. Aust Dent J 2002;47:123–30.

[6] Wyatt C. Elderly Canadians residing in long-term care hospitals. Part 2. Dental caries status. CDA J 2002;68:359–63.

[7] Saub R, Evans R. Dental needs of elderly hostel residents of inner Melbourne. Aust Dent J 2001;46:198–202.

[8] Frenkl H, Harvey I, Newcombe R. Oral health care in nursing home residence in Avon. Gerodontology 2000;17:33–8.

[9] Weyant R, Hobbins N, Niessen L, et al. Oral health status of a long term care veteran population. Community Dent Oral Epidemiol 1993;21:227–33.

[10] Thomson W. Dental caries experience in older people over time: what can the large cohort studies tell us? Br Dent J 2004;196:89–92.

[11] Fure S. Ten-year incidence of tooth loss and dental caries in elderly Swedish individuals. Caries Res 2003;37:462–9.

[12] Chalmers J, Carter K, Spencer A. Caries incidence and increments in community living older adults with and without dementia. Gerodontology 2002;19:80–94.

[13] Thomson W, Spencer A, Slade G, et al. Is medication a risk factor for dental caries among older people? Community Dent Oral Epidemiol 2002;30:224–32.

[14] Luan W, Baelum V, Fejerskob O, et al. Ten year incidence of dental caries in adult and elderly Chinese. Caries Res 2000;34:205–13.

[15] Drake C, Beck J, Lawrence H, et al. Three-year coronal caries incidents and risk factors in North Carolina elderly. Caries Res 1997;31:1–7.

[16] Lawrence H, Hunt R, Beck J, et al. Five-year incidence rates and intra-oral distribution of root caries among community dwelling older adults. Caries Res 1996;30:169–79.

[17] Hand J, Hunt R, Beck J. Incidence of coronal and root caries in an older adult population. J Pub Health Dent 1988;48:14–9.

[18] Chestnut I, Binnie V, Taylor M. Reasons for tooth extraction in Scotland. J Dent 2000;28: 295–7.

[19] Slade G, Spencer A, Locker D, et al. Variations in the social impact of oral conditions among older adults in South Australia, Ontario, and North Carolina. J Dent Res 1996;75:1439–50.

[20] Lin B, Taylor G, Allen D, et al. Dental caries in older adults with diabetes mellitus. Spec Care Dentist 1999;19:8–14.

[21] Yoshihara A, Hanada N, Miyazaki H. Association between serum albumin and root caries in community-dwelling older adults. J Dent Res 2003;82:218–22.

[22] Maupome G, Gullion C, White B, et al. Oral disorders and chronic systemic diseases in very old adults living in institutions. Spec Care Dentist 2003;23:199–208.

[23] Mandel I. Oral infections: impact on human health, well-being, and health-care costs. Compend Contin Educ Dent 2002;23:403–6.

[24] Gilbert G, Duncan R, Dolan T, et al. Twenty-four months of root caries among a diverse group of adults. Caries Res 2001;35:366–75.

[25] Saunders R, Handelman S. Effects of hyposalivatory medications on salivary flow rates and dental caries in adults age 65 and older. Spec Care Dentist 1992;12:116–21.

[26] Morse D, Holm-Pedersen P, Holm-Pedersen J, et al. Prosthetic crowns and other clinical risk indicators of caries among old-old Swedish adults: findings from the Keohs project. Kungsholmen Elders Oral Health Study. Gerodontology 2002;19:73–9.

[27] Jepson N, Moynihan P, Kelly P, et al. Caries incidents following restoration of shortened lower dental arches in a randomized controlled trial. Br Dent J 2001;191:140–4.

[28] Avlund K, Holm-Pedersen P, Morse D, et al. Tooth loss and caries prevalence in very old Swedish people: the relationship to cognitive function and functional ability. Gerodontology 2004;21:17–26.

[29] Steele JG, Sheiham A, Marcenes W, et al. National Diet and Nutrition Survey: people aged 65 and over. London: HM Stationary Office; 1998.

[30] Shah N, Sundaram KR. Impact of sociodemographic variables, oral hygiene practices, oral habits and diet on dental caries experience of Indian elderly: a community based study. Gerodontology 2004;21:43–50.

[31] Vargas C, Yellowitz J, Hayes K. Oral health status of older rural adults in the United States. J Am Dent Assoc 2003;134:479–86.

[32] Kurzon MEJ, Preston AJ. Risk groups: nursing bottle caries/caries in the elderly. Caries Res 2004;38(Suppl 1):24–33.

[33] Featherstone J, Adair S, Anderson M, et al. Caries management by risk assessment: consensus statement, April 2002. Journal of the California Dental Association 2003;31:257–69.

[34] Glassman P, Anderson M, Jacobsen P, et al. Practical protocols for the prevention of dental disease in community settings for people with special needs: the protocol. Spec Care Dentist 2003;23:160–4.

[35] Kaltjens H, van Der Hoeven J, Schaeken J. Etiology and prevention of root caries. Ned Tijdschr Tandhellk 1992;99:217–9.

[36] Jensen M, Kohout F. The effect of a fluorided dentifrice on root and coronal caries in an older population. J Am Dent Assoc 1998;117:829–32.

[37] Davies R. The rational use of oral care products in the elderly. Clin Oral Investig 2003;8:2–5.

[38] Kelly M, Steele J, Nuttall N, et al. Adult dental health survey: oral health in the United Kingdom 1998. London: HM Stationery Office; 2000.

[39] Stephen K, Creanor S, Russell J, et al. A 3 year oral health dose-response study of sodium monofluorophosphate dentifrices with and without zinc citrate: anti-caries results. Community Dent Oral Epidemiol 1998;16:321–5.

[40] Baysan A, Lynch E, Ellwood R, et al. Reversal of primary root caries using dentifrices containing 5000 and 1100 ppm fluoride. Caries Res 2001;35:41–6.

[41] Sjogern K, Birkhed D. Factors related to fluoride retention after use of fluoride. Caries Res 1993;27:474–7.

[42] Ripa L, Leske G, Forte F, et al. Effect of a 0.05% NaF rinse on coronal and root caries in adults. Gerodontology 1987;6:131–6.

[43] Fure S, Gahnberg L, Birkhed D. A comparison of four home care fluoride programs on the caries incidence in the elderly. Gerodontology 1998;15:51–8.

[44] Wallace M, Retief D, Bradley L. The 48 month increments of root caries in an urban population of older adults participating in a preventive dental program. J Public Health Dent 1993;53:133–7.

[45] Saunders R, Handelman S. Coronal and root decay in institutionalized older adults. N Y State Dent J 1991;57:25–8.

[46] Billings R, Meyerowitz C, Featherstone J, et al. Retention of topical fluoride in the mouths of xerostomic subjects. Caries Res 1988;22:306–10.

[47] Seppa L, Leppanen T, Hausen H. Fluoride varnish vs. acidulated phosphate fluoride gel. A three year clinical trial. Caries Res 1995;29:327–30.

[48] Hawkins R, Locker D, Noble J, et al. Prevention. Part 7: Professionally applied topical fluorides for caries prevention. Br Dent J 2003;195:313–7.

[49] Weintraub J. Fluoride varnish for caries prevention: comparisons with other preventive agents and other recommendations for a community-based protocol. Spec Care Dentist 2003;23:180–6.

[50] Schaeken M, Keltjens H, van der Hoeven J. The effect of fluoride and chlorhexidine on the microflora of dental root surfaces and progression of root surface caries. J Dent Res 1991;70: 150–3.

[51] Johnson G, Almqvist H. Non-invasive management of superficial root caries lesions in disabled and infirm patients. Gerodontology 2003;20:9–14.

[52] Brailsford S, Fiske J, Gilbert S, et al. The effects of the combination of chlorhexidine/thimol and fluoride containing varnishes on the severity of root caries lesions in frail institutionalized elderly people. J Dent 2002;30:319–24.

[53] Powell V, Leroux B, Martin J, et al. Identification of adult populations at high risk for dental caries using a computerized database and patient records: a pilot project. J Public Health Dent 2000;60:82–4.

[54] Bondestam O, Ghanberg L, Sund M, et al. Effect of chlorhexidine gel treatment on the prevalence of the mutans streptococci and lactobacilli in patients with impaired saliva rate. Spec Care Dent 1996;16:123–7.

[55] Sarner B, Lingstrom P, Birkhed D. Fluoride release From NaF and AmF impregnated toothpicks and dental flosses in vitro and in vivo. Acta Odontol Scand 2003;61: 289–96.

[56] Wallman C, Birkhed D. Effect of chlorhexidine varnish and gel on mutans streptococci in margins of restorations in adults. Caries Res 2002;36:360–5.

[57] Anderson M. Chlorhexidine and xylitol gum in caries prevention. Spec Care Dentist 2003;23: 173–6.

[58] Pihlanto-Leppala A, Soderling E, Makinen K. Expulsion mechanism of xylitol 5-phosphate in Streptococcus mutans. Scand J Dent Res 1990;98:112–9.

[59] Soderling E, Isokangas P, Tenovuo J, et al. Long-term xylitol consumption and mutans streptococci in plaque and saliva. Caries Res 1991;25:153–7.

[60] Simons D, Brailsford S, Kidd E, et al. The effect of chlorhexidine/xylitol chewing gum on the plaque and gingival indices of elderly occupants in residential homes. J Clin Periodontol 2001;28:101–5.

[61] Hilderbrandt G, Sparks B. Maintaining mutans streptococci suppression with xylitol chewing gum. J Am Dent Assoc 2000;131:909–16.

[62] Gaffar A, Blake-Haskins J, Sullivan R, et al. Effects of a xylitol/NaF dentifrice in vivo. Int Dent J 1998;48:32–9.

[63] Wyatt C, MacEntee M. Dental caries in chronically disabled elders. Spec Care Dentist 1997; 17:196–202.

[64] Powell V, Leroux B, Martin J, et al. Identification of adult population at high risk for dental caries using a computerized database and patient records: a pilot project. J Public Health Dent 2000;60:82–4.

[65] Anusavice K. Dental caries: risk assessment and treatment solutions for an elderly population. Compend Contin Educ Dent 2002;23:12–20.

[66] Leak J. Clinical decision making for caries management in root surfaces. J Dent Educ 2001; 65:1147–53.

[67] Holmes J. Clinical reversal of root caries using ozone: double-blind, randomized, controlled 18-month trial. Gerodontology 2003;20:106–14.

[68] Ericson D, Zimmerman M, Raber H, et al. Clinical evaluation of efficacy and safety of a new method for chemo-mechanical removal of caries: a multi-center study. Caries Res 1999;33: 171–7.

[69] Rafique S, Fiske J, Banerjee A. Clinical trial of an air-abrasion/chemo-mechanical operative procedure for the restorative treatment of dental patients. Caries Res 2003;37:360–4.

[70] Cole B, Welbury R. The atraumatic restorative treatment (ART) technique: does it have a place in everyday practice? Dent Update 2000;27:118–20.

[71] Hu J, Ley Smales R, Yip K. Restoration of teeth with more-viscous glass ionomer cements following radiation-induced caries. Int Dent J 2002;52:445–8.

[72] Hadley J, Young D, Eversole L, et al. A laser powered hydrokinetic system for caries removal and cavity preparation. J Am Dent Assoc 2000;131:777–85.

[73] Ajdic D, McShan W, McLaughlin R, et al. Genome sequence of *Streptococcus mutans* UA159, a cariogenic dental pathogen. Proc Natl Acad Science 2002;99(22):144434–9.

[74] Quivey R, Fozo E. Finding the hole in the defenses of cavity-creating microbes. University of Rochester Medical Center News Archives. June 25, 2004.

ELSEVIER
SAUNDERS

THE DENTAL
CLINICS
OF NORTH AMERICA

Dent Clin N Am 49 (2005) 309–326

Salivary Hypofunction and Xerostomia: Diagnosis and Treatment

Jane C. Atkinson, DDS[a],*, Margaret Grisius, DMD[b],
Ward Massey, BDS, PhD[c]

[a]Comprehensive Care and Therapeutics, University of Maryland Dental School,
666 West Baltimore Street, 3E-32, Baltimore, MD 21201-1586, USA
[b]Gene Therapy and Therapeutics Branch, National Institute of Dental and Craniofacial
Research, 10 Center Drive, Room 1N-113, MSC 1190, Bethesda, MD 20892-1190, USA
[c]Restorative Dentistry and Biomaterials Science, Harvard School of Dental Medicine,
188 Longwood Avenue, Boston, MA 02115, USA

Saliva plays a central role in the maintenance of oral homeostasis. The complex mixture of proteins, glycoproteins, mucins, and ions helps prevent dental caries, promotes remineralization of early carious lesions, buffers acids generated by oral bacteria, and prevents other types of oral infections [1]. Proteins such as salivary peroxidase, lysozyme, and lactoferrin are antibacterial and limit the growth of cariogenic bacteria. The film of salivary mucins on the teeth and mucosal surfaces is believed to protect these oral structures from wear. Histatins, a family of salivary proteins, have potent antifungal properties that limit the growth of oral yeast. These salivary components, in conjunction with the mucosal tissues, form part of the innate immune system that continually protects the human body from infection. The oral cavity also is protected by secretory immunoglobulins A and M, which are produced locally by B cells within the salivary glands. These antibodies include those with specificity against oral cariogenic bacteria. Other evidence suggests that saliva may be important in protecting and healing the esophagus. It neutralizes acid that protects the esophagus from damage after gastric reflux and contains growth factors that could stimulate epithelial growth to promote healing [2].

When salivary volume is reduced significantly, patients are at risk for serious oral complications. Several clinical studies have demonstrated that caries and salivary flow rates are associated. Reports that root caries rates

---

* Corresponding author.
E-mail address: jatkinso@mail.nih.gov (J.C. Atkinson).

0011-8532/05/$ - see front matter © 2005 Elsevier Inc. All rights reserved.
doi:10.1016/j.cden.2004.10.002

are inversely proportional to flow rates and to the use of medications with xerostomic effects [3,4] and that adults with a whole stimulated salivary flow of less than 1.0 mL/min were more likely to lose teeth [5] provide evidence that saliva is crucial to the prevention of dental caries. However, an evidence-based review published in 2001 concluded that no evidence linked a "missing salivary element" to the development of caries in humans [6]. The only clear association between caries and saliva was between the amount of caries and the volume of salivary flow.

Another sequela of low salivary flow rates is an increase in oral infections such as candidiasis. Saliva contains histatins, a family of low molecular weight proteins that both inhibit and kill candidal organisms. Lysozyme also contributes to the antifungal properties of saliva, and recent evidence suggests that saliva collected from elders has a reduced ability to inhibit attachment of *Candida* to surfaces [7]. Fungal load in the mouth is inversely proportional to stimulated salivary gland flow rates [8,9], and overt candidal infections occur more often in patients with decreased salivary flow [10].

Saliva participates in the formation of the initial food bolus, begins digestion, and aids the swallowing process. Other complications associated with severe reductions in salivary flow rates include swallowing difficulties [11], decreases or alterations in taste [12], and aggravation of conditions such as gastroesophageal reflux disease [13]. Decreases in taste and difficulties in swallowing can force elders to alter food choices [14].

Prevalence of xerostomia and decreased salivary flow in elders

Many elder groups have been studied to determine their frequency of dry mouth complaints and their salivary flow rates. To appreciate these studies, it is first necessary to understand two related concepts. First, complaints of dry mouth (or xerostomia) may not reflect reduced salivary function and may instead reflect dehydration or other systemic conditions. Therefore, studies that only examine the complaints of dry mouth will not reflect the true risk for oral diseases in the population. Second, it is very difficult to determine values for normal salivary function, because normal values vary considerably, and large patient groups must be compared to make meaningful conclusions about changes in salivary flow rates.

Several healthy patient cohorts were examined in the 1980s and 1990s to determine whether salivary gland function declined with age. Some studies suggest that there are small declines in the salivary function of women with age [15], whereas earlier studies found no effect [16]. Although salivary function generally is conserved in healthy, unmedicated persons aged more than 65 years, these individuals constitute a very small percentage of this age group. Other studies suggest that salivary flow rates in elders are related to the number of medications they take on a regular basis [17,18], the number of systemic disorders they report, and the length of time for which they consume the drugs [19].

Medications and salivary hypofunction

Medication use is believed to be the most common reason for reduction of salivary flow in older individuals. This effect is primarily mediated through medications' anticholinergic actions or their effect on fluid balance. Many diuretics, antihypertensives, antihistamines, sedatives, opioid analgesics, tricyclic antidepressives, and major antipsychotics will reduce flow. It is estimated that 50% of the noninstitutionalized adult population in the United States takes at least one prescription medication, and those using the highest number of medications are women aged 65 years or older [20]. In one study of women aged more than 65 years, 12% took at least 10 medications, and 23% took at least five prescription drugs. Polypharmacy in elders increases the risk for adverse side effects [21], including oral dryness. Evidence that medication usage by the aged increased during the 1990s comes from a Finnish study [22] that assessed changes in medication use among community-dwelling persons aged 64 years or older in 1990 to 1991 (n = 1131) and 1998 to 1999 (n = 1197). Among those surveyed, 78% in 1990 to 1991 and 88% in 1998 to 1999 used prescription drugs. The number of medications per person increased from 3.1 to 3.8, and polypharmacy (concomitant use of more than five medications) increased from 19% to 25%. Other evidence suggests that the salivary glands of older persons may be more susceptible to medications with anticholinergic effects and that there is a reduced "reserve" in the glands of older individuals [23,24].

Several studies of nursing home patients have documented a high incidence (up to 63%) of dry mouth complaints and decreased salivary flow rates in a large percentage of the residents (Table 1) [14,25–27]. Xerostomia is also a frequent complaint of the community-dwelling population over 65 years of age, with an estimated prevalence of 11% to 57% (see Table 1) [11,17,28–32]. Both salivary flow rates and complaints of oral dryness are related to medication use in the elderly (see Table 1). Data from these studies also suggest that elderly women may have more dryness complaints than men, that oral dryness causes swallowing and chewing difficulties, and that tooth loss is related to salivary flow rates.

Autoimmune diseases

Sjögren's syndrome (SS) is an autoimmune exocrinopathy that primarily affects salivary and lacrimal glands. Although case reports appeared in the literature before 1930, the syndrome is named for the Swedish ophthalmologist Henrik Sjögren, who first described a group of women with xerostomia, rheumatoid arthritis, and a type of eye dryness termed keratoconjunctivitis sicca. Further studies by Bloch et al [33] defined primary and secondary forms. Patients may have primary Sjögren's syndrome (only salivary and lacrimal gland involvement) or salivary or lacrimal gland dysfunction in association with another major connective

Table 1
Representative studies of xerostomia complaints and salivary flow rates in elders

Author	Residence of subjects: hospital, resident facilities, or community dwelling	Number of elderly subjects	Findings
Thorelius et al (1988) [25]	Resident facilities	149	11% had very low stimulated whole flow; number of drugs taken inversely correlated with flow; women more likely to have dryness complaints.
Handelman et al (1989) [26]	Resident facilities	157	61% reported oral dryness; number of drugs taken inversely correlated with stimulated whole salivary flows.
Loesche (1995) [14]	Hospital, resident, and community dwelling	123 resident homes or community; 218 outpatient controls; 132 long-term VA facilities; 81 hospitalized	Stimulated flow rates lower in those complaining of oral dryness; 55% using at least one xerogenic medication; 86% xerogenic drug use by those in long-term facilities. Patients with xerostomia had more difficulty chewing and swallowing and avoided certain foods. Ipratropium, oxybutynin, triazolam, amitriptyline, and tropical triamcinolone were related to oral dryness.
Pajukoski et al (2001) [27]	Hospital and community dwelling	175 hospitalized; 252 community-dwelling	63% of hospitalized subjects had oral dryness versus 57% of community-subjects. In all patients, psychiatric drug use was the strongest predictive factor for dry mouth.

Österberg et al (1984) [28]	Community dwelling	973 for interview; subset of 58 men and 51 women for salivary flow rates	Women more likely to have dryness complaints; dryness complaints related to number of medications taken and to consumption of diuretics and anticholinergic medications. Salivary flow rates negatively correlated to tooth loss.
Ben-Aryeh et al (1985) [29]	Community dwelling	259	28% had oral dryness; anticholinergic medications, sympatholytic agents, and diuretics used more frequently by those with oral dryness.
Sreebny et al (1988) [17]	Outpatients	185 subjects aged 55 or older (subset of 529)	Oral dryness related to number of medications taken; 29% of entire group had complaints of oral dryness.
Gilbert et al (1993) [30]	Community dwelling	600	39% had oral dryness complaints; dryness complaints associated with xerogenic medication use; 10% of those with dryness complaints had difficulty swallowing.
Locker (1995) [32]	Community dwelling	Longitudinal study of 611 patients aged 50 or older	Oral dryness complaints in the group increased from 15% to 29.5% in 3 years. Those reporting poor health were more likely to have oral dryness. Onset of oral dryness and eating complaints may be associated.

tissue disease, such as rheumatoid arthritis, systemic lupus erythematosus, scleroderma, or primary biliary cirrhosis. Most academic health centers have adopted the modified European criteria for the diagnosis of Sjögren's syndrome [34], and estimates of its prevalence range between 0.5% and 1.5% worldwide [35].

The hallmarks of Sjögren's syndrome are intense, activated plasmolymphocytic infiltrates of the lacrimal and salivary glands [36], high-titered autoantibodies, hypergammaglobulinemia, and a loss of secretory function by the salivary and lacrimal glands [37]. The loss of saliva and tears can produce severe oral and ocular dryness and associated diseases. Other patient complaints include difficulty in eating, speaking, and swallowing and burning or itching of the eyes and mouth. Over 90% of patients with primary SS are female, often in their fifth decade of life when diagnosed. However, it is not uncommon to diagnose the syndrome in children, young women, and patients aged 65 to 80 years.

Primary SS is a systemic disease [37]. Infiltrating lymphocytes can compromise many organ systems, producing what are known as extra-glandular manifestations of SS. Most serious is malignant lymphoma, which is estimated to occur 20 to 30 times more frequently in these patients. A longitudinal study of patients with primary SS found that those with low complement fraction 4 in their serum had a significantly increased mortality [37]. Other studies in recent years have examined quality of life issues in SS patients. Fatigue is a common complaint, as well as an increased incidence of depressed mood, reduced sense of well-being, and impaired vitality [38,39]. Treatment for Sjögren's syndrome consists of preventive and palliative treatments (see further discussion). Unfortunately, clinical trials with systemic anti-inflammatory agents and other immunosuppressives have not been successful to date in this patient group, but several trials are ongoing. Topical anti-inflammatory agents, such as cyclosporine eye preparations and an alpha-interferon oral lozenge [40], have had some positive results in clinical trials.

Radiation therapy

It is estimated that 28,000 patients per year in the United States have high-dose, external beam radiation to eradicate a tumor of the head and neck region. New cases are concentrated in patients aged 50 years or older. Approximately 90% of the tumors are squamous cell carcinomas, and treatment consists of surgery or external beam radiotherapy. Unfortunately, the salivary gland tissue that is included in the field of radiation suffers a permanent loss of function, usually within the first 2 weeks of fractionated radiation treatment [41]. The reasons for the high radio-sensitivity of salivary tissues are not well understood, but at present the best option for treatment is to avoid irradiating some salivary tissue (see later discussion of treatment). The known mechanisms of radiation damage and other treatment issues for the head and neck radiation patient were recently reviewed [41]. The internal radiation agent I_{131} (radioactive iodine) also can damage salivary tissue, although usually not to the same extent as external radiation [42].

Other diseases

Several other diseases have been associated with reduced salivary function or xerostomia. These include hypertension (both treated and untreated), diabetes, depression, and dementia of the Alzheimer's type.

Hypertension was associated with decreased flow rates and complaints of oral dryness in very early studies. It was hypothesized that the salivary glands of individuals with hypertension received inadequate parasympathetic stimulation [43]. Recent studies suggest that medications, rather than hypertension, depress salivary flow in hypertensive individuals [44,45], but these studies were conducted with small patient groups. The antisalivation properties of clonidine have been studied in clinical trials [45], whereas beta-blocking agents alter the protein composition of saliva [46]. Antihypertensive agents such as diuretics are frequently associated with complaints of oral dryness (see Table 1).

Patients with poorly controlled diabetes were found to have decreased salivary flow rates in a study by Chavez et al [47]. Patients with dementia of the Alzheimer's type [48] and untreated depression also are reported to have decreased salivary flow [49].

Treatment

Treatments for salivary gland diseases vary according to their cause, and potential treatments for diseased or nonfunctional salivary glands are active areas of research (Box 1). However, many recommended treatments have not been tested in well-designed clinical trials [50]. Currently available treatments for salivary gland hypofunction and xerostomia can be classified into four major categories: (1) prevention, (2) symptomatic treatment, (3) local or topical salivary stimulants, and (4) systemic therapies.

Prevention

Preventive measures must be emphasized with every patient who has decreased salivary function. Frequent dental examinations are essential. For patients receiving radiation therapy, strategies are available to limit salivary gland exposure. Radiation stents can be fabricated to shield the ipsilateral side when unilateral radiation treatment is required. Another method of limiting radiation to salivary glands is conformal and intensity-modulated irradiation (IMRT). This technique, first reported by Eisbruch et al [51], targets the lesion while sparing the major salivary glands from radiation. After 1 year, patients treated using IMRT had fewer xerostomia complaints,

Box 1. Guidelines for treatment of patients with decreased salivary function

I. Establish the cause of the decreased salivary flow rate.
  a. Does the patient have Sjögren's syndrome?
  b. Is the patient taking multiple medications daily (more than five) or a medication with significant anticholinergic effects?
  c. Is there a history of internal or external radiation treatment?
  d. Does the patient have multiple systemic illnesses?

II. Take preventive measures.
  a. Remind the patient that the use of sugared products throughout the day to stimulate flow will significantly increase dental caries.
  b. Prescribe a supplemental fluoride that is appropriate for patient's caries risk.
  c. Recall the patient every 3–4 months until caries control is achieved.
  d. Discuss with the physician the feasibility of altering the type of medication to one with fewer anticholinergic effects or of changing the time of day the medication is taken.
  e. Discuss with the patient's oncologist the possibility of using radiology techniques that spare one or more salivary glands from radiation.

III. Administer symptomatic treatment.
  a. Encourage the patient to sip water throughout the day.
  b. Recommend salivary substitutes or coating agents.
  c. Recommend humidifying the environment.

IV. Promote salivary stimulation.
  a. Advise the patient to use *sugarless* candies, mints, or gum to stimulate flow.
  b. Prescribe pilocarpine or cevimeline for 2 months if not medically contraindicated. Discontinue if there is no improvement of signs or symptoms after 2 months.

V. Plan restorative treatment.
  a. Early diagnosis of caries and intervention is essential.
  b. Select a direct resin restorative material based on its mechanical and fluoride-releasing properties.
  c. Make every effort to "do no harm." In some cases, it is acceptable to do less rather than more.
  d. Before providing extensive restorative treatment, determine that the patient can maintain it.

a higher quality of life, and less loss of total parotid gland function than patients treated with conventional radiotherapy [51,52].

Amifostine is an oxygen scavenger that may protect salivary glands from free-radical damage during radiation therapy. It has a broad spectrum of cyto-protective and radio-protective functions. Amifostine is reported to protect the salivary glands and reduce xerostomia during head and neck radiation therapy. However, it requires intravenous drug administration before each radiation treatment and has associated side effects [53–56].

Patients with reduced salivary flow also have an increased incidence of oral fungal infections and salivary gland infections. Sugarless antifungal agents such as nystatin powder and clotrimazole vaginal troches can be used to treat infections without increasing the caries risk. In addition, any intraoral acrylic prosthesis used by an infected patient must be soaked in an antifungal agent. Patients should be encouraged to maintain an adequate fluid intake and remain hydrated to prevent bacterial infections of the glands. Milking the salivary glands daily by gentle massage, sucking on sugarless candies, and wiping the oral cavity with glycerine swabs will help prevent mucous plug formation and salivary gland infections.

Modification of a patient's medication regimen can reduce the degree of medication-induced dryness complaints. Substituting different medications with fewer anticholinergic effects can reduce oral dryness. For example, patients report fewer side effects with the medication donepezil than with other medications used to treat memory loss associated with Alzheimer's disease [57]. Serotonin-specific reuptake inhibitors are reported to cause xerostomia less frequently than do tricyclic antidepressants [58,59]. Olanzapine is an antipsychotic medication that has markedly reduced xerostomia side effects but similar efficacy when compared with chlorpromazine [60]. Another method of reducing xerostomia is to alter the time of day when medications are taken. Salivary flow declines at night. Taking a medication that reduces flow and causes xerostomia in the morning or dividing medication doses when possible may improve oral comfort.

Symptomatic treatment

Water is the most important treatment for symptoms of dry mouth. Sipping water throughout the day keeps the oral mucosa hydrated and clears debris from the mouth. Sipping water during meals aids in chewing, swallowing, and taste perception. Caffeine-containing beverages should be avoided. The geriatric population is more susceptible to dehydration and should be reminded to drink water on a regular basis. Using a room humidifier increases environmental humidity and may improve patients' oral comfort, resulting in more restful sleep.

Many over-the-counter products are available for the symptomatic relief of oral dryness. Patients should be advised not to use products containing alcohol or strong flavors, which may irritate the mucosa. Patients should avoid sugar-containing products because of their increased susceptibility to dental caries. Artificial salivas can provide some relief for patients with low salivary gland function. Most available in the United States contain carboxymethylcellulose, whereas mucin-based products are available in Europe. Saliva substitutes and the oral lubricant Oralbalance (Biotene, Rancho Dominguez, California) [61] may increase patient comfort, but these substitutes have not been shown to reduce the risk for caries or other oral infections associated with reduced salivary output.

Salivary stimulation with local or topical regimens

Sugar-free candies, gums, and mints can stimulate salivary flow. The combination of chewing and taste can provide significant relief for patients who have some remaining salivary gland function. Xylitol is a low-calorie sugar product in gums and mints that suppresses growth of cariogenic streptococci and reduces caries [62]. Electrical stimulation has been used as a treatment for xerostomia. Low-voltage electrical stimulation was shown many years ago to increase salivary output, but only limited evidence of its efficacy exists. Recently, Domingo [63] investigated the effects of electrostimulation with a hand-held transcutaneous electrical nerve stimulator and found that the unit improved parotid salivary flow in 6 of 18 patients.

Systemic stimulation

Although several agents have been proposed as systemic sialogogues to treat salivary gland dysfunction and xerostomia, most have not been tested in randomized clinical trials with objective measures of salivary function. Only two secretagogues, pilocarpine and cevimeline, have been approved by the US Food and Drug Administration.

Pilocarpine hydrochloride is derived from the *Pilocarpus jaborandi* plant. Field workers in Brazil would chew this plant while working to increase salivary flow, prompting Coutinho, a Brazilian physician, to suggest *P jaborandi* as a treatment for dry mouth. Pilocarpine is a parasympathetic agent that functions as a nonspecific muscarinic agonist with mild beta-adrenergic activity. This alkaloid causes pharmacologic stimulation of exocrine glands. Pilocarpine acts by stimulating functioning salivary gland tissue; consequently, patients with little functioning salivary gland parenchyma may have no improvement of symptoms with its use. However, patients with severe salivary gland destruction may still report improvement of symptoms with the medication. Therefore, a 2-month trial of pilocarpine is recommended. If the patient does not feel any improvement in xerostomia or the physician sees no improvement in the clinical signs of salivary hypofunction, it should be discontinued.

Pilocarpine is the most widely studied systemic sialogogue. In 1991, Fox et al [64] published a double-blind, placebo-controlled study of 39 patients with salivary hypofunction (mostly from SS and postradiotherapy to the head and neck). A dose of 5 mg three times a day reduced complaints of oral dryness and increased unstimulated flow rates. Multicenter trials found similar results for patients after head and neck radiation and those with SS [65]. Gotrick et al [66] found pilocarpine effective in the treatment of opioid-induced xerostomia, suggesting that it may be beneficial for the treatment of some medication-induced oral dryness.

The usual oral dosage for pilocarpine is 5 to 10 mg three times per day. The initial recommended dose is 5 mg three times per day, which can be increased up to 30 mg/d depending on response and tolerance. The onset of action is 30 minutes, and the duration of action is approximately 2 to 3 hours. Common side effects include gastrointestinal upset, sweating, tachycardia, bradycardia, increased pulmonary secretions, increased smooth muscle tone, and blurred vision. Contraindications include gall bladder disease, angle closure glaucoma, and renal colic. Risk to the patient must be considered when administering to patients with heart disease, asthma, angina pectoris, chronic bronchitis, chronic obstructive pulmonary disease, or a history of myocardial infarction. Pilocarpine may interact with various medications, including beta adrenergic antagonists and other parasympathomimetic drugs, and could antagonize the therapeutic anticholinergic effects of medications such as oxybutynin.

Cevimeline is a cholinergic agonist with selectivity for two of the five known muscarinic receptors. Studies suggest that these receptors are the primary mediators of salivation. In 2000, the US Food and Drug Administration approved the drug for the treatment of autoimmune-associated xerostomia. The effectiveness of this medication is limited in that it only stimulates remaining functioning salivary gland tissue. Unlike pilocarpine, which is a nonselective muscarinic agonist, cevimeline selectively binds to the M1 and M3 receptors [67]. Although fewer cardiac and respiratory side effects should be experienced with cevimeline, those experienced in clinical trials are similar to those of pilocarpine. Cevimeline is only taken three times daily, because its duration of action is longer than that of pilocarpine [68]. The same precautions apply to use of cevimeline and pilocarpine. Patients with uncontrolled asthma, cardiac disease, or angle closure glaucoma should not take the drug.

Restorative considerations in the dry mouth patient

Two crucial principles should be observed when dealing with the restorative needs of the patient with decreased salivary flow or xerostomia. The first of these is the necessity for early diagnosis and intervention in caries development [69]. Any patient at high risk for the development of dental caries requires frequent recall. Patients should be maintained at a 3-month recall frequency until the level of caries risk and activity falls to moderate and then placed on 6-month recall until the risk falls to a low level. At recall appointments, dental hard tissues should be examined closely for primary and secondary caries in a dry field, using magnification and caries detection dyes where appropriate.

The rate of caries development in even the highest-risk patient will usually allow for some monitoring of early smooth-surface nonproximal lesions. Where patient compliance is good and the lesion is visible, accessible, in enamel, and noncavitated, an arresting treatment with a concentrated fluoride varnish (such as 5% sodium fluoride containing fluoride at 25,000 ppm) and monitoring at 3-month recall is a viable option [70]. If cavitation, even superficial, is detected or suspected or the lesion is proximal or in a high-risk area of the tooth, plaque entrapment and progression should be assumed in the dry mouth patient [71]. Restoration with a fluoride-releasing restorative material is the preferred treatment [72].

The second principle to apply to the restorative needs of the patient with complaints of oral dryness is "do no harm." Where restorative treatment is necessary to restore carious tooth structure, careful selection of the technique and restorative material is extremely important. Conservative cavity preparation techniques and adhesive material systems should be used wherever possible to avoid unnecessary removal of sound tooth structure and achieve retention. Several aspects of each restorative material should be considered before selection: retentive mechanism, tendency to protect remaining tooth structure, prevention of secondary caries, tendency to assist remineralization of tooth structure, longevity under functional load, and aesthetics.

Materials currently available can be divided broadly into direct and indirect materials, based on their method of clinical placement. Direct restoratives are so named because they are deformable when mixed and placed. After placement, they can be molded into an appropriate form before they set. These materials vary in their physical properties and ability to support remaining tooth structure [73]. The direct restoratives include composite resins, polyacid-modified composite resins, resin-modified glass ionomers, conventional glass ionomers, and dental amalgam. Indirect restorative materials are formed in the laboratory, and the finished restoration is luted into the preparation. Consequently, preparation of a cavity form without undercuts is required. This group of materials includes indirect composite inlays, onlays, and veneers, ceramic inlays, onlays, and veneers, and gold and porcelain-fused-to-gold full and partial veneers. Because a common path of withdrawal is needed for these materials, the preparations are far less conservative of tooth structure than those required for direct restoratives.

Keeping these factors in mind, one observes that a direct plastic restorative material is the obvious choice for the small to moderately sized carious lesion in a patient with dry mouth. Removal of tooth structure can also be kept to a minimum through the use of materials with adhesive capabilities. The fact that these restorations can be readily and inexpensively added to, modified, repaired, or replaced makes a direct restorative the obvious choice for the dry mouth patient in whom caries activity is unpredictable or difficult to monitor. It is also wise to use direct materials until the caries risk and activity levels have stabilized.

Where extensive damage to tooth structure exists, adhesive techniques can be used in conjunction with direct and indirect materials to optimize marginal seal and minimize unnecessary removal of tooth structure for retention of the restoration. Restoration margins should be placed in areas that facilitate monitoring and cleaning whenever possible. Fluoride-releasing luting cements such as a glass ionomer, which also possess good film-thickness properties, should be used when possible with indirect restoratives [74].

When extensive treatment is provided to a dry mouth patient, it must be predetermined that the patient can maintain the restored dentition. In theory, all restorative options should be available, but, in reality, the oral and systemic health of the patient often dictates modification of treatment.

Direct restorative materials for patients with reduced salivary flow

Matching the properties of restorative materials to patients' needs for oral and systemic health is the key to prognosis. For patients with some salivary flow, the selection of fluoride-releasing restorative materials is advantageous because of their ability both to prevent secondary caries and to assist in remineralization [75–77].

Fluoride-releasing restorative materials can be classified into four major categories on the basis of their physical, chemical, and clinical properties [71]. At one end of the continuum lie the conventional (chemical set) glass ionomers; at the other, the fluoride-releasing composite resins. The polyacid-modified composite resins (compomers) are more closely aligned with resin composites, whereas resin-modified glass ionomers behave similarly to conventional glass ionomers [78].

Resin composites have superior mechanical and aesthetic properties and greater wear resistance than the other materials listed. Some resin composites have the ability to release fluoride, albeit in far smaller amounts than glass ionomer restoratives. Glass ionomers have inherent adhesion to dentin and release comparatively high amounts of fluoride (sufficient to remineralize enamel but not dentin), but their mechanical properties and wear resistance are inferior. Resin-modified glass ionomers have improved aesthetics but in other respects behave like glass ionomers and hence should not be used on load-bearing areas [78].

Compomers behave more like fluoride-releasing composite resins because they contain more resin than glass ionomers. In vitro, it has been noted that the adhesive systems used by composite resins and compomers prevent the uptake of fluoride released from the restorative material by tooth structure [79]. The clinical significance of this finding is still unknown. Fluoride released from glass ionomer restorative materials can be measured in whole saliva in vivo, and its incorporation into tooth structure can be measured by microbiopsy techniques [80,81]. However, the fluoride release in tooth structure has been found to be localized to within 1 mm of the restoration margin [82]. Fluoride released from conventional glass ionomer restoratives has been measured over time and found to be at its highest level 1 to 2 days after placement [83]. It then drops substantially but is still detectable up to 1 year after placement. [84]. The lower salivary pH values often found in severe dry mouth patients appear to accelerate fluoride release [85]. This effect is hypothesized to result from erosion of the alumino-fluorosilicate glass particle surface.

Probably the most important feature of fluoride-releasing restorative materials in the high-caries-risk dry mouth patient is not their initial fluoride release but their capacity to be "recharged" with fluoride from external sources [86]. Conventional glass ionomers show the greatest fluoride "recharge" capacity, followed by compomers and resin-modified glass ionomers. Fluoride-releasing composite resins do not exhibit this property [87]. Fluoride may be replenished with toothpastes, rinses, or solutions. Frequent application is necessary, because fluoride release on "recharge" has been shown to be of short duration (approximately 1 day) [87]. Daily topical application is therefore recommended. Acidulated phosphate fluoride products should not be used, because they cause etching and degradation of the restoration surface of glass ionomers, resin-modified glass ionomers, and compomers [88]. Neutral sodium fluoride gels, pastes, and rinses are the easiest means of "recharge" in dry mouth patients.

Theoretically, it should be possible to control all new caries through the "recharge" of fluoride-releasing restorative materials. However, when the salivary pH stays below 4.5 for prolonged periods (as it can in a dry mouth patient), the potential for remineralization is inhibited. The most common fluoride products that can be applied topically for "recharge" are sodium fluoride, stannous fluoride, and sodium monofluorophosphate. The vehicle most commonly used is a dentifrice containing fluoride at around 1000 ppm. Neutral sodium fluoride gels containing fluoride at around 10,000 ppm or neutral sodium fluoride rinses containing fluoride from 100 to 1000 ppm can also be applied daily [89].

Summary

Salivary gland hypofunction and complaints of xerostomia are common in elderly patients, irrespective of their living situation. Medication use is frequently related to dry mouth symptoms and reductions in salivary flow rates. Patients with reduced salivary flow are at increased risk for caries, oral fungal infections, swallowing problems, and diminished or altered taste. Oral health care providers should institute aggressive preventive measures and recommend palliative care for patients with significant reduction in salivary gland function. The systemic agents pilocarpine and cevimeline may help selected patients. Selective use of fluoride-releasing restorative materials and conservative treatment plans are recommended for this patient group.

References

[1] Van Nieuw Amerongen A, Bolscher JG, Veerman EC. Salivary proteins: protective and diagnostic value in cariology? Caries Res 2004;38(3):247–51.

[2] Pedersen AM, Bardow A, Jensen SB, et al. Saliva and gastrointestinal functions of taste, mastication, swallowing and digestion. Oral Dis 2002;8(3):117–29.

[3] Papas AS, Joshi A, MacDonald SL, et al. Caries prevalence in xerostomic individuals. J Can Dent Assoc 1993;59(2):171–4, 177–9.

[4] Kitamura M, Kiyak HA, Mulligan K. Predictors of root caries in the elderly. Community Dent Oral Epidemiol 1986;14(1):34–8.

[5] Caplan DJ, Hunt RJ. Salivary flow and risk of tooth loss in an elderly population. Community Dent Oral Epidemiol 1996;24(1):68–71.

[6] Leone CW, Oppenheim FG. Physical and chemical aspects of saliva as indicators of risk for dental caries in humans. J Dent Educ 2001;65(10):1054–62.

[7] Kamagata-Kiyoura Y, Abe S, Yamaguchi H, et al. Reduced activity of Candida detachment factors in the saliva of the elderly. J Infect Chemother 2004;10(1):59–61.

[8] Radfar L, Shea Y, Fischer SH, et al. Fungal load and candidiasis in Sjögren's syndrome. Oral Surg Oral Med Oral Pathol Oral Radiol Endod 2003;96(3):283–7.

[9] Wahlin YB. Salivary secretion rate, yeast cells, and oral candidiasis in patients with acute leukemia. Oral Surg Oral Med Oral Pathol 1991;71(6):689–95.

[10] Navazesh M, Wood GJ, Brightman VJ. Relationship between salivary flow rates and Candida albicans counts. Oral Surg Oral Med Oral Pathol Oral Radiol Endod 1995;80(3): 284–8.

[11] Rudney JD, Ji Z, Larson CJ. The prediction of saliva swallowing frequency in humans from estimates of salivary flow rate and the volume of saliva swallowed. Arch Oral Biol 1995;40(6): 507–12.

[12] Ikebe K, Sajima H, Kobayashi S, et al. Association of salivary flow rate with oral function in a sample of community-dwelling older adults in Japan. Oral Surg Oral Med Oral Pathol Oral Radiol Endod 2002;94(2):184–90.

[13] Valdez IH, Fox PC. Interactions of the salivary and gastrointestinal systems. I. The role of saliva in digestion. Dig Dis 1991;9(3):125–32.

[14] Loesche WJ, Bromberg J, Terpenning MS, et al. Xerostomia, xerogenic medications and food avoidances in selected geriatric groups. J Am Geriatr Soc 1995;43(4):401–7.

[15] Ghezzi EM, Wagner-Lange LA, Schork MA, et al. Longitudinal influence of age, menopause, hormone replacement therapy, and other medications on parotid flow rates in healthy women. J Gerontol A Biol Sci Med Sci 2000;55(1):M34–42.

[16] Baum BJ. Salivary gland fluid secretion during aging. J Am Geriatr Soc 1989;37(5):453–8.

[17] Sreebny L, Valdini A, Yu A. Xerostomia. Part II: Relationship to nonoral symptoms, drugs and diseases. Oral Surg Oral Med Oral Pathol 1989;68(4):419–27.

[18] Wu AJ, Ship JA. A characterization of major salivary gland flow rates in the presence of medications and systemic diseases. Oral Surg Oral Med Oral Pathol Oral Radiol Endod 1993;76(3):301–6.

[19] Navazesh M, Brightman VJ, Pogoda JM. Relationship of medical status, medications, and salivary flow rates in adults of different ages. Oral Surg Oral Med Oral Pathol Oral Radiol Endod 1996;81(2):172–6.

[20] Kaufman DW, Kelly JP, Rosenberg L, et al. Recent patterns of medication use in the ambulatory adult population of the United States: the Slone survey. JAMA 2002;287(3): 337–44.

[21] Bressler R, Bahl JJ. Principles of drug therapy for the elderly patient. Mayo Clin Proc 2003; 78(12):1564–77.

[22] Linjakumpu T, Hartikainen S, Klaukka T, et al. Use of medications and polypharmacy are increasing among the elderly. J Clin Epidemiol 2002;55:809–17.

[23] Ghezzi EM, Ship JA. Aging and secretory reserve capacity of major salivary glands. J Dent Res 2003;82(10):844–8.

[24] Wu AJ, Baum BJ, Ship JA. Extended stimulated parotid and submandibular secretion in a healthy young and old population. J Gerontol A Biol Sci Med Sci 1995;50A:M45–8.

[25] Thorselius I, Emilson CG, Österberg T. Salivary conditions and drug consumption in older age groups of elderly Swedish individuals. Gerodontics 1988;4(2):66–70.

[26] Handelman SL, Baric JM, Saunders RH, et al. Hyposalivatory drug use, whole stimulated salivary flow, and mouth dryness in older, long-term care residents. Spec Care Dentist 1989; 9(1):12–8.

[27] Pajukoski H, Meurman JH, Halonen P, et al. Prevalence of subjective dry mouth and burning mouth in hospitalized elderly patients and outpatients in relation to saliva, medication, and systemic diseases. Oral Surg Oral Med Oral Pathol Oral Radiol Endod 2001; 92(6):641–9.

[28] Österberg T, Landahl S, Hedegård B. Salivary flow, saliva, pH and buffering capacity in 70-year-old men and women. J Oral Rehab 1984;11(2):157–70.

[29] Ben-Aryeh H, Miron D, Berdicevsky I, et al. Xerostomia in the elderly: prevalence, diagnosis, complications and treatment. Gerodontology 1985;4(2):77–82.

[30] Gilbert GH, Heft MW, Duncan RP. Mouth dryness as reported by older Floridians. Community Dent Oral Epidemiol 1993;21(6):390–7.

[31] Thomson WM, Chalmers JM, Spencer AJ, et al. Medication and dry mouth: findings from a cohort study of older people. J Public Health Dent 2000;60(1):12–20.

[32] Locker D. Xerostomia in older adults: a longitudinal study. Gerodontology 1995;12(1): 18–25.

[33] Bloch KJ, Buchanan WW, Wohl MJ, et al. Sjögren's syndrome: a clinical, pathological and serological study of sixty-two cases. Medicine (Baltimore) 1965;44:187–231.

[34] Vitali C, Bombardieri S, Jonsson R, et al. Classification criteria for Sjögren's syndrome: a revised version of the European criteria proposed by the American-European Consensus Group. Ann Rheum Dis 2002;61(6):554–8.

[35] Dafni UG, Tzioufas AG, Staikos P, et al. Prevalence of Sjögren's syndrome in a closed rural community. Ann Rheum Dis 1997;56(9):521–5.

[36] Daniels TE. Labial salivary gland biopsy in Sjögren's syndrome. Assessment as a diagnostic criterion in 362 suspected cases. Arthritis Rheum 1984;27(2):147–56.

[37] Skopouli FN, Dafni U, Ioannidis JP. Clinical evolution and morbidity and mortality of primary Sjögren's syndrome. Semin Arthritis Rheum 2000;29(5):296–304.

[38] Strombeck B, Ekdahl C, Manthorpe R, et al. Health-related quality of life in primary Sjögren's syndrome, rheumatoid arthritis, and fibromyalgia compared to normal population using SF-36. Scand J Rheumatol 2000;29(1):20–8.

[39] Valtysdottir ST, Gudbjornsson B, Lindqvist U, et al. Anxiety and depression in patients with primary Sjögren's syndrome. J Rheumatol 2000;27(1):165–9.

[40] Ship JA, Fox PC, Michalek JE, et al. Treatment of primary Sjögren's syndrome with low-dose natural human interferon-alpha administered by the oral mucosal route: a phase II clinical trial. IFN Protocol Study Group. J Interferon Cytokine Res 1999;19(8):943–51.

[41] Vissink A, Burlage FR, Spijkervet FK, et al. Prevention and treatment of the consequences of head and neck radiotherapy. Crit Rev Oral Biol Med 2003;14(3):213–25.

[42] Caglar M, Tuncel M, Alpar R. Scintigraphic evaluation of salivary gland dysfunction in patients with thyroid cancer after radioiodine treatment. Clin Nucl Med 2002;27(11): 767–71.

[43] Rahn KH, van Baak M, van Hooff M, et al. Studies on salivary flow in borderline hypertension. J Hypertens Suppl 1983;1(2):77–8.

[44] Streckfus CF, Wu AJ, Ship JA, et al. Comparison of stimulated parotid salivary gland flow rates in normotensive and hypertensive persons. Oral Surg Oral Med Oral Pathol 1994;77(6): 615–9.

[45] Nederfors T, Dahlof C. Effects on salivary flow rate and composition of withdrawal of and re-exposure to the beta 1–selective antagonist metoprolol in a hypertensive patient population. Eur J Oral Sci 1996;104(3):262–8.

[46] Gretler DD, Gramelspacher GP, Fumo MT, et al. Influence of diuretic therapy on the clonidine suppression test. J Clin Pharmacol 1991;31(5):448–54.

[47] Chavez EM, Taylor GW, Borrell LN, et al. Salivary function and glycemic control in older persons with diabetes. Oral Surg Oral Med Oral Pathol Oral Radiol Endod 2000;89(3): 305–11.

[48] Ship JA, DeCarli C, Friedland RP, et al. Diminished submandibular salivary flow in dementia of the Alzheimer type. J Gerontol 1990;45(2):M61–6.

[49] Palmai G, Blackwell B, Maxwell AE, et al. Patterns of salivary flow in depressive illness and during treatment. Br J Psychiatry 1967;113:1297–308.

[50] Brennan MT, Shariff G, Lockhart PB, et al. Treatment of xerostomia: a systematic review of therapeutic trials. Dent Clin North Am 2002;46(4):847–56.

[51] Eisbruch A, Ship JA, Dawson LA, et al. Salivary gland sparing and improved target irradiation by conformal and intensity modulated irradiation of head and neck cancer. World J Surg 2003;27(7):832–7.

[52] Parlimant MB, Scrimger RA, Anderson SG, et al. Preservation of oral health–related quality of life and salivary flow rates after inverse-planned intensity-modulated radiotherapy (IMRT) for head and neck cancer. Int J Radiat Oncol Biol Phys 2004;58(3):663–73.

[53] Mehta M. Amifostine and combined-modality therapeutic approaches. Semin Oncol 1999; 26(2):95–101.

[54] Wasserman T. Radioprotective effects of amifostine. Semin Oncol 1999;26(2):34–6.

[55] Taylor SE, Miller EG. Preemptive pharmacologic intervention in radiation-induced salivary dysfunction. Proc Soc Exp Biol Med 1999;221(1):14–26.

[56] Rades D, Fehlauer F, Bajrovic A, et al. Serious adverse effects of amifostine during radiotherapy in head and neck cancer patients. Radiother Oncol 2004;70(3):261–4.

[57] Jacobsen FM, Comas-Diaz L. Donepezil for psychotropic-induced memory loss. J Clin Psychiatry 1999;60(10):497–504.

[58] Hunter KD, Wilson WS. The effects of antidepressant drugs on salivary flow and content of sodium and potassium ions in human parotid saliva. Arch Oral Biol 1995;40(11):983–9.

[59] Trindade E, Menon D, Topfer LA, et al. Adverse effects associated with selective serotonin reuptake inhibitors and tricyclic antidepressants. A meta analysis. CMAJ 1998;159(10): 1245–52.

[60] Conley RR, Tamminga CA, Bartko JJ, et al. Olanzapine compared with chlorpromazine in treatment-resistant schizophrenia. Am J Psychiatry 1998;155(7):914–20.

[61] Alves MB, Motta AC, Messina WC, et al. Saliva substitute in xerostomic patients with primary Sjögren's syndrome: a single-blind trial. Quintessence Int 2004;35(5):392–6.

[62] Van Loveren C. Sugar alcohols: what is the evidence for caries-preventive and caries-therapeutic effects? Caries Res 2004;38(3):286–93.

[63] Domingo DL. The effects of electrostimulation on saliva production in postradiation head and neck cancer patients. Oral Surg Oral Med Oral Pathol Oral Radiol Endod 2004;97(4):464.

[64] Fox PC, Atkinson JC, Macynski AA, et al. Pilocarpine treatment of salivary gland hypofunction and dry mouth (xerostomia). Arch Intern Med 1991;151(6):1149–52.

[65] Atkinson JC, Baum BJ. Salivary enhancers. J Dent Educ 2001;65(10):1096–101.

[66] Gotrick B, Akerman S, Ericson D, et al. Oral pilocarpine for treatment of opiod-induced oral dryness in healthy adults. J Dent Res 2004;83(5):393–7.

[67] Shiozawa A. Cevimeline hydrochloride hydrate (Saligren capsules 30 mg): a review of its pharmacologic profiles and clinical potential in xerostomia. Nippon Yakurigaku Zasshi 2002;120(4):253–8.

[68] Fox RI. Cevimeline, a muscarinic M1 and M3 agonist, in the treatment of Sjögren's syndrome. Adv Exp Med Biol 2002;506(Pt B):1107–16.

[69] Atkinson JC, Wu AJ. Salivary gland dysfunction: causes, symptoms and treatment. J Am Dent Assoc 1994;125:409–16.

[70] Jensen MF, Kohout F. The effect of a fluoride dentifrice on root and coronal caries in an older population. J Am Dent Assoc 1988;117:829–32.

[71] Featherstone JDB. Fluoride, remineralization and root caries. Am J Dent 1994;7:279.

[72] Haveman CN, Redding SW. Dental management and treatment of xerostomic patients. Tex Dent J 1998;115:43–56.

[73] Burgess JO, Norling B, Ong J, et al. Directly placed esthetic restorative materials. Compend Contin Educ Dent 1996;17:731–48.

[74] Rezk-Lega F, Ogaard B, Rolla G. Availability of fluoride from glass ionomer luting cements in human saliva. Scand J Dent Res 1991;99:60–3.

[75] Benelli EM, Serra MC, Rodrigues AL Jr, et al. In-situ anti-cariogenic potential of glass-ionomer cement. Caries Res 1993;27:280–4.

[76] Tyas MJ. Cariostatic effect of glass-ionomer cement—a 5 year study. Aust Dent J 1991;36: 236–9.

[77] Xu X, Burgess JO, Turpin-Mair JS. Fluoride release and recharge of fluoride releasing restorative materials [Abstract 431]. J Dent Res 1999;78:159.

[78] Forsten L, Paunio IK. Fluoride release by silicate cements and resin composites. Scand J Dent Res 1972;80:515–9.

[79] Burgess JO, Norling BK, Summitt JB. Resin ionomer restorative materials: the new generation. J Esthet Dent 1994;6:207–15.

[80] Burkett L, Burgess JO, Chan DCN, et al. Fluoride release of glass ionomers coated and not coated with adhesive [Abstract 1242]. J Dent Res 1993;72:258.

[81] Halgreen A, Oliveby A, Twetman S. Fluoride concentration in plaque adjacent to orthodontic appliances retained with glass ionomer cement. Caries Res 1993;27:51–4.

[82] Phillips RW, Swartz ML. Effect of certain restorative materials on the solubility of enamel. J Am Dent Assoc 1957;54:623–6.

[83] Tantibironj D, Douglas WH, Versluis A. Inhibitive effect of a resin modified glass ionomer cement on remote artificial caries. Caries Res 1997;31:275–80.

[84] Hatibovic-Hofman S, Koch G. Fluoride release from glass ionomer cement in-vivo and in-vitro. Swed Dent J 1991;15:253–8.

[85] Alvarez AN, Burgess JO, Chan DCN. Short-term fluoride release of six ionomers—recharged, coated and abraded [Abstract 260]. J Dent Res 1994;73:134.

[86] Cranfield M, Kuhn A, Winter GB. Factors relating to the rate of fluoride release from glass ionomer cement. J Dent 1982;10:333–41.

[87] Daamen JJM, Buijs MJ, ten Cate JM. Uptake and release of fluoride by saliva coated glass ionomer cement. Caries Res 1996;30:454–7.

[88] El-Badrawy WA, McComb D. Effect of home use fluoride gels on resin modified glass ionomer cement. Oper Dent 1998;23:2–9.

[89] Forsten L. Short-term and long-term fluoride release from glass ionomer and other fluoride containing materials in-vitro. Scand J Dent Res 1990;98:179–85.

ELSEVIER
SAUNDERS

THE DENTAL
CLINICS
OF NORTH AMERICA

Dent Clin N Am 49 (2005) 327–342

Derangement, Osteoarthritis, and Rheumatoid Arthritis of the Temporomandibular Joint: Implications, Diagnosis, and Management

Jack S. Broussard, Jr, DDS

University of Southern California, School of Dentistry, Oral Health Center,
3151 South Hoover Street, Los Angeles, CA 90089-7792, USA

The prevalence of deterioration of both function and form from "wear and tear" in the load-bearing joints of the body increases with aging. Wear and tear deterioration of a joint is called osteoarthritis. Sometimes the dysfunction is a discal derangement problem and does not involve deterioration of the surfaces of the joint. Whether the dysfunction is osteoarthritis or derangement, when it is isolated to one joint, the origin is generally traumatic. When the dysfunction is polyarthritic in nature, the agents of crystal deposition, autoimmunity, Lyme disease infection, and idiopathic causation are evoked.

Polyjoint arthritic disease is extremely common in the human population, with the highest prevalence in the elderly. Polyjoint osteoarthritis is by far the most common of the rheumatic diseases affecting an estimated 20.7 million Americans and is responsible for over 7 million patient visits per year [1–3]. When all of the arthritic diseases are added together, over 70 million United States citizens (one in three adults) report a rheumatic disease [4]. In the group of those 75 years or older, a majority reports having arthritis. As might be expected given this high prevalence, the social and economic impact of rheumatic diseases taxes our health care systems. Adults over the age of 65 have more patient visits for these diseases than any other age group [5]. In addition to clear-cut rheumatologic disease, more than 100 medical conditions affect the muscles, tendons, and joints and are classified as musculoskeletal-related diseases. It is hypothesized that approximately 33% of the United States population demonstrates signs and symptoms of

E-mail address: jbroussa@usc.edu

0011-8532/05/$ - see front matter © 2005 Elsevier Inc. All rights reserved.
doi:10.1016/j.cden.2004.10.003
dental.theclinics.com

musculoskeletal disease [5,6]. Moreover, $118.5 billion per year has been spent by United States citizens on the care of musculoskeletal diseases [4,6]. Over $86.2 billion is spent annually on rheumatic diseases [4]. The percentage cost of the United States gross national product used to treat musculoskeletal disease has increased each decade since the 1960s. When these diseases are severe, mobility and functional limitations cause increases in work loss, disability, use of nursing care, and premature retirement. Musculoskeletal disorders are second only to heart diseases as a cause of work disability. Work-loss costs associated with rheumatic diseases account for 50% to 76.5% of all indirect costs [4]. As the older population increases in number and longevity, these costs will continue to rise.

The good news is that the temporomandibular joint (TMJ) is less likely to show aging-related deterioration than are other major body joints, perhaps because the TMJ is less of a load-bearing joint than the knee, shoulder, or spine. Moreover, the prevalence of TMJ signs and symptoms decreases with age. In adult nonpatient populations, the prevalence of at least one sign of temporomandibular disorders (TMD) ranges from 40% to 50% [7–10]. Limited jaw opening may occur in 5% [11]. With the exception of limited opening, which has a slightly higher prevalence in the elderly, the prevalence of jaw pain and TMJ clicking appears to be stable across adulthood, then inexplicably decrease in the population aged more than 65 years. Matsuka et al [12] investigated the prevalence of signs and symptoms of TMD in Japan. They examined 672 individuals (304 men and 368 women between ages of 20 and 92) selected randomly in Okayama City, Japan. They reported that, although TMD signs and symptoms were common in all age groups, they were less numerous in the older age group. Notably, they also reported that clicking was higher in the younger adults, whereas crepitation increased significantly in the oldest age group.

It is perplexing that the elderly do not exhibit more clinical symptoms of joint pain when we consider that the TMJ shows increased morphologic changes with aging, suggesting increased deterioration [13,14]. For example, one postmortem study of elderly cadavers found that 91% of joints examined had morphologic changes, including osteoarthritic change [14]. This article reviews normal anatomy and function of the TMJ, derangements, localized osteoarthritis (OA), generalized or polyjoint OA, and rheumatoid arthritis as they relate to the TMJ and the elderly.

Normal and age-related changes in temporomandibular joint anatomy and physiology

The TMJ is a complex synovial joint. It is the only joint in the human body where the condyle slides completely out of its socket yet is not considered dislocated. This joint is unique in that it can undergo not only hinge movement but also extensive translational or sliding movement. It contains a meniscus composed of dense fibrous connective tissue; the temporal and condylar articular surfaces are also covered with fibrocarti-lage, rather than the more typical hyaline cartilage seen in other joints [15,16]. Synovial fluid lubricates the joint and the loading of the articular fibrocartilage, and subchondral bone causes chondrocytes in the articular cartilage to synthesize and secrete collagen, proteoglycans, and other proteins necessary for cartilage and subchondral bone repair [17–21]. Proteoglycan molecules consist of a protein core with negatively charged glycosaminoglycan side chains composed of keratin sulfate and chondroitin sulfate. Aggregates of proteoglycans are linked to a core of hyaluronic acid, allowing the binding of large numbers of water molecules inside this complex molecule. Compression of the cartilage releases this fluid, which is recaptured as compression is removed [20]. This fluid movement allows cartilage to undergo reversible deformations.

Why does the TMJ exhibit such a high prevalence of wear-and-tear–related problems with aging? One explanation is that the interposing disk between the condyle and the temporal component of the joint is damaged or displaced. However, many patients develop joint arthritic changes in-dependent of disk displacement. Certainly crystal deposits (eg, gout and pseudogout) inside the joint, Lyme disease, and autoimmunity reactions also explain joint-surface deterioration. The first two conditions (ie, crystal deposition arthritis and Lyme disease) are not discussed in this article; autoimmunity-related arthritis is covered in the section on rheumatoid arthritis. Another, and perhaps the most important, reason joints break down and become arthritic involves changes in the frictional interface between the condyle, disk, and temporal components of the TMJ.

As in all synovial joints, the fibrocartilage and TMJ disk are largely acellular and are maintained in health and repaired and lubricated by the synovial fluid in the joint. High load or loading that occurs with inadequate lubrication results in a surface breakdown, leading to OA [22]. Aging has been reported to induce articular cartilage thinning in synovial joints: the cartilage actually changes color (from white to a dull yellow) [23]. In addition, the fluid that lubricates and protects the joint surface changes with age. Aging is accompanied by reduced accumulation of this synovial fluid and the synthesis of smaller proteoglycans, which hold less water and exhibit reduced compressive ability and more breakdown in the surface of the joint. This process increases keratin sulfate and reduces chondroitin sulfate content in the synovial fluid. These changes, partially caused by the decrease in water content that accompanies aging and a change in cartilage pro-teoglycan, are considered one of the earliest signs of articular cartilage loss in OA. Nakayama et al [24] examined normal synovial fluid and measured the concentrations of chondroitin 6-sulfate (C6S), chondroitin 4-sulfate (C4S), and hyaluronic acid in healthy subjects of different ages. The subjects were 82 healthy volunteers ranging in age from 20 to 79 years. They found that the concentrations of CS and hyaluronic acid varied with age. Their values were highest between 20 and 30 years of age and thereafter showed a tendency to decrease. The ratio of C6S to C4S was significantly lower in the group aged 60 to 70 years when compared with the 20- to 30-year-old group. In fact, multiple regression analysis demonstrated that age correlated strongly with the C6S concentration and the C6S to C4S ratio (ratio = −0.521 and −0.617, respectively).

The oddity of the aged TMJ is that, even though the joint shows clear signs of deterioration, it is not highly painful in most of the patients who have arthritic alteration of the joint. It is possible that TMJ deterioration changes are better tolerated (less painful) in the elderly than in younger patients. In fact, research has suggested that the degree of inflammation cartilage damage induces in the elderly is inferior to that caused by the same insult and injury to the joint of a young patient. This concept of reduced degradation is based on the work of DeGroot et al [25], who reported on an age-related decrease in the susceptibility of human articular cartilage to matrix metalloproteinase–mediated degradation. Specifically, they looked at the effect of age-related accumulation of advanced glycation end products (AGEs) on cartilage. They found that, the more AGEs were accumulated, the less susceptible the cartilage was to proteolytic degradation by matrix metalloproteinases present in synovial fluid in both OA and rheumatoid arthritis patients. The joint deterioration changes seen in the elderly, which have developed slowly and progressively across a lifetime, may also be better tolerated than problems due to acute injury in younger patients. A change in nociceptive physiology may even occur in the elderly.

Local temporomandibular joint disk dysfunction in the elderly

Although disk derangement of the TMJ is more common in the 20- to 50-year-old population, the elderly have their share of dysfunction (clicking and locking). When an elderly patient develops new-onset TMJ clicking, the first order of business is to rule out osteoarthritic disease as the underlying cause. If no OA changes are evident on the imaging of the joint, then education about the need to avoid this frictional event during function is essential to reducing the likelihood of progression to a more serious deterioration of the joint. This approach is called avoidance therapy and has three components. First, the patient is shown how to limit the degree of jaw opening and protrusion, thus stopping translation and TMJ clicking. Second, the patient is informed that chewing on the same side as the click usually helps to avoid it and is provided with a chewable substance (eg, gum) so they can attest, under the physician's observation, that this is so. Third, the patient is informed that a dietary change to small bites and soft food will be necessary to avoid the click. Strict avoidance of all clicking and all gum chewing is required. It should be clearly understood that this approach will not stop clicking, only reduce the number of times the disk is jammed between the condyle and eminence, thus reducing wear and tear on these tissues.

In the elderly patient who presents with a jaw locked open, manipulation of the jaw is necessary to achieve a closure of the opening. Depending on how long the jaw has been locked, the manipulation of the jaw can usually be performed without adjunctive medications (antispasmodics). Assuming the mandible is locking in a wide-open position, this manipulation involves holding the mandible with both hands, placing the thumb on the back molars of the lower jaw and the fingers under the mandible on each side. The manipulation is performed by pushing down on the mandible with the thumbs while pulling up on the anterior portion of the mandible with the fingers. When successful, this manipulation allows the condyle to move down and then back, so that it can then move posteriorly to the TMJ eminence. If manual manipulation alone is not successful, the next step is to sedate the patient with a short-acting benzodiazepine. This medication can be delivered orally (if the patient can swallow) or intravenously (if he or she cannot swallow or if haste is needed in the reduction process). Once reasonable sedation is achieved, the previously described manipulation is usually easier to perform.

In those cases where the open locking problem has been reduced but has become a recurrent event, a thorough history and examination of the TMJ with tomographic or MR imaging should be completed. If these films show no osseous abnormality or substantial disk derangement, the primary therapy is to avoid wide opening to prevent more recurrences of the open locking. If, however, a substantial articulator surface or discal disease is present, the primary treatment for a mechanical derangement of the TMJ is arthroscopic surgery to achieve a thorough lavage and stretching of the TMJ.

Local temporomandibular joint arthritis in the elderly

Localized OA is characterized by focal degeneration of joint cartilage with osseous erosion and sclerosis and sometimes osteophyte formation occurring at the joint margins [26]. It is considered a disease of the bone, cartilage, and supporting tissues and results from both mechanical and biologic events that destabilize the normal coupling of degradation and synthesis of articular cartilage and subchondral bone [22]. Localized OA is usually thought to be traumatic in nature (either macrotrauma or repetitive microtrauma) but may also be due to a rare infective arthritic disease. When an elderly patient comes to a dentist's office with a complaint of jaw pain, the most likely diagnosis is localized arthritis (assuming the patient does not exhibit polyjoint arthritic disease). The arthritis can usually be discovered with palpation, auscultation, and radiographic examination of the joint. Occasionally, the jaw joint pain is related to a disk derangement of the jaw (clicking, locking, or dislocation), but OA is the more prevalent problem among the elderly. Dulcic et al [27] examined the frequency of internal derangement of the TMJ in elderly individuals. They examined the TMJ of 96 elderly subjects (mean age 76) and reported that a clinical diagnosis of internal derangement of the TMJ was present in only 9.3% of the subjects. By contrast, about 20% of a younger population (ages 20–50) typically exhibit noticeable symptoms of internal derangement.

As mentioned earlier, clicking and locking do not increase among the elderly, but localized OA does. In a 2003 study based on a European population, Gillette and Tarricone [28] reported that the prevalence of OA is approximately 12% for subjects between 25 and 50 years of age but reaches as high as 95% in the subset of patients over 60 years of age. Fortunately, osteoarthritic changes in the TMJs of the elderly population are much less prevalent than the above data for all body sites might suggest. Specifically, Hiltunen et al [29] reported on a random sample (N = 88) of elderly subjects between the ages of 76 and 86 years living in Helsinki. The most frequent radiographic finding in the TMJ was flattening of the articular surface, indicating OA, which occurred in 17% of the population.

Still, assuming that 17% of the population over 65 have TMJ osteoarthritic change and 9.3% have internal derangement, this is a large group of patients. It is likely that as many as 50% of those with radiographic change have at least a mild-to-moderate degree of pain and dysfunction in their jaws. Aging in and of itself is not thought to cause OA, but if a combination of several age-related changes occurs in the same individual, OA will result. Specifically, forceful repetitive function (eg, bruxism) or disk displacement, along with synovial fluid alterations of the TMJ, will predispose the elderly individual to OA.

Treatment of localized osteoarthritis and derangement in the elderly

When joint pain symptoms occur and management is required, the principles governing treatment of the TMJ are no different from those used to treat other body joints with painful OA. Treatment always begins with nonpharmacologic therapy, which includes patient education, rest, and physical therapy, including the use of occlusal appliances (when tooth clenching or an unstable bite is evident). Education should be directed toward reducing stressful jaw function (eg, chewing hard foods) and reducing or eliminating aggravating factors, such as teeth clenching, opening wide, and gum chewing. One consistent feature of arthritic disease management that applies to both TMJ derangement and TMJ arthritis is that the patient must be taught about the chronic nature of the disease. It is sometimes difficult for patients to accept that the displaced disk in their jaw joint cannot be put back in place or that the damaged joint tissues cannot be repaired or replaced. Depending on the medical propaganda to which patients have been exposed, they may have unrealistic treatment expectations, which can lead to frustration and depression.

Physical therapy for TMJ OA usually consists of teaching the patients how to perform jaw exercises and apply heat or ice packs to the jaw. Two primary jaw/tongue posture exercises are recommended. First and foremost is the "N" position exercise, which involves placing the jaw and tongue in the position achieved when saying the letter "N" and holding it for a count of 10. The patient is instructed to perform this exercise hourly each day (or 12 times a day). The goal is to put and hold the jaw in the most relaxed jaw position where the teeth are apart and the lips not touching. Once patients' initial pain symptoms are shown to be reduced, they can proceed to the next exercise, called the jaw hinge exercise. The patient is instructed (with use of mirror feedback) to move the jaw carefully in a strict hinge motion to a point about 15 mm open and then close it again. This motion promotes synovial fluid movement without any translation of the condyle. The motion is usually performed 15 times on a 2- to 3-hour schedule, or six times a day.

Although the N-position and hinge exercises help reduce strain on the joint, it is also advisable to apply 20 minutes of heat therapy (hot towels or a moist heating pad) to the sorest muscles. Heat helps to reduce pain and stiffness by relaxing aching muscles and increasing circulation to the area. Finally, nonopioid analgesics and nonsteroidal anti-inflammatory drugs can be helpful. (For more information see article on prescriptions and over-the-counter medications for arthritis in the elderly elsewhere in this issue.)

Corticosteroid injections help with any inflammatory TMJ pain problem that is unresponsive to the usual treatments. This approach may be an early treatment intervention in patients with gastritis, gastro-esophageal reflux disorder, or other indications for not using a nonsteroidal anti-inflammatory medication. When indicated, a corticosteroid intra-articular injection using one of several different corticosteroids is appropriate; a common one is triamcinelone [30,31]. The usual amount of medication injected in a single jaw joint is 10 to 20 mg. The injection is targeted to the superior joint space, and the corticosteroid is usually mixed with an equal amount of local anesthetic to make the joint injection more comfortable. After the injection, it is wise to recommend ice packs as needed and a completely soft diet for 48 hours until the injection has an effect on the inflammation. The general guideline is that the TMJ should not be injected more than twice in a 12-month period.

Vallon et al [32] examined the possibility of long-term adverse effects of repeated corticosteroid injections on the TMJ in patients with rheumatoid arthritis (RA). They performed a long-term (12-year) follow-up of 21 patients with RA and symptomatic TMJs who received either an intra-articular injection of a steroid (n = 11) or a local anesthetic agent (n = 10). Fourteen patients who were available for long-term follow-up reported no pain from the TMJ. Radiographic follow-up examination was performed on 12 patients, and all but 4 of the 24 joints had structural bone changes. Interestingly, the magnitude and prevalence of change was no different in the two groups. The investigators concluded that the chances of long-term progression of joint destruction for the steroid-injected and non–steroid-injected joints were equivalent in this patient group with RA. Presumably these results can be generalized to osteoarthritic disease in the TMJ.

For patients who have only a transient response to the corticosteroids, hyaluronic acid injections have been used with moderate success for new-onset OA with crepitation. Intra-articular hyaluronic acid injection can provide symptomatic relief for several months. Two approved drugs currently exist: Synvisic and Hyalgan. These medications are given in a series of three injections, 1 month apart, and are currently approved for knee joints [33,34]. They have been approved for OA of the knee and are also helpful for TMJ pain and dysfunction. One of the first studies of the use of hyaluronate in the TMJ was performed over a decade ago by Bertolami et al [35], who studied 121 patients at three test sites using a randomized, double-blind, placebo-controlled experimental design. Patients were selected on the basis of a confirmed diagnosis of degenerative joint disease (DJD), reducing displaced disc (DDR), or nonreducing displaced disc (DDN), along with nonresponsiveness to nonsurgical therapies and a severe jaw dysfunction according to several measures. Subjects received either a unilateral upper joint space injection of 1% sodium hyaluronate (HA) in physiologic saline or a United States Pharmacopia physiologic saline injection. The researchers reported no differences for DJD and only minor difference for DDN. However, for DDR they found a statistically significant within-group and between-group improvement throughout the 6-month test period. More recently, Shi et al [36] have evaluated the effect of HA on TMJ degenerative and derangement disorders using a prospective, randomized, controlled clinical trial in 67 subjects (12 men, 51 women). They provided HA injections in the upper compartments of the involved TMJs, with 35 patients receiving 6 mg of 1% HA and 28 receiving 12.5 mg of prednisolone. The protocol in this study included three to four injections over a 2-month treatment period. The investigators concluded that the intra-articular injection of HA is effective and safe for the treatment of TMJ degenerative disorders, with mild adverse reactions.

Topical creams (eg, capsaicin or nonsteroidal anti-inflammatory drugs [NSAIDs]) have been described as being helpful if the patient does not tolerate oral medications and does not want an injection-based therapy. Many products are sold over the counter to help patients with arthritis pain. However, the experimental data for transdermal therapy in arthritis are weak. For example, Winocur et al [37] examined the effect of topical application of capsaicin on localized pain in the TMJ area. They conducted a randomized, double-blind, placebo-controlled study in 30 patients suffering from unilateral pain in the TMJ area. Patients received either 0.025% capsaicin cream or its vehicle and were instructed to apply the cream to the painful TMJ area four times daily for 4 weeks. Capsaicin cream produced no statistically significant difference in the outcome measures when compared with placebo. This general result was supported by another, more recent study by Myrer et al [38], who examined the effects of a topical analgesic and placebo in treatment of chronic knee pain. They conducted a double-blind, randomized, placebo-controlled clinical trial in 46 men and women with chronic knee pain. Testing took place before treatment and after 21 and 35 days of treatment. Although both groups experienced improved pain scores, there were no differences between groups over the treatment period for any of the dependent variables.

Another topical medication (transdermal lidocaine patch) has become available for neuropathic pain. The effect of this new patch on OA was recently evaluated by Burch et al [39]. Specifically, they looked at the effectiveness of the lidocaine patch 5% on pain, stiffness, and function in OA pain patients in a prospective, multicenter, open-label effectiveness trial. The authors concluded that the lidocaine patch 5% appears effective as an add-on therapy for OA pain. They recommended the use of up to four patches, changed every 24 hours, to provide effective analgesia without anesthesia and to reduce stiffness and disability and improve quality of life in polyjoint arthritis patients, particularly those who have responded incompletely to prior medication therapy. This approach has the advantage of offering an effective topical analgesic option for OA with a minimal risk of systemic toxicity or drug interactions. Obviously, controlled clinical trials are needed to confirm the efficacy and safety of lidocaine patch 5% therapy.

Finally, arthrocentesis-based lavage is useful for TMJs with limited mobility but is controversial as a treatment for joint pain without joint hypomobility. The primary goal of this procedure is to mobilize the TMJ; it involves washing the joint with saline solution and conducting manual manipulation of the jaw when it is anesthetized. It plays a role primarily in those patients who do not respond to pharmacologic treatment and present with limited opening. The long-term benefits of arthrocentesis lavage are unknown; only limited good-quality comparative therapy studies have been done. Moreover, there are no data on the efficacy of arthrocentesis in the elderly TMJ. Nitzan and Price [40] looked at the use of arthrocentesis for the treatment of osteoarthritic TMJs. Specifically, they examined 36 patient records in a retrospective fashion. The patients were 29 women and 7 men (aged 16 to 54 years) presenting with 38 dysfunctional joints that exhibited OA and had not responded to conservative treatment. The authors reassessed the patients after arthrocentesis, at a time point varying from 6 to 62 months. They reported that, of the 38 OA TMJs treated with arthrocentesis, 26 joints reacted favorably to the treatment. The authors even stated that in many instances the osteoarthritic TMJs returned to a healthy functional state. Emshoff and Rudisch [41] looked more closely at who benefited from an arthrocentesis procedure. They evaluated 29 TMJ pain patients with a diagnosis of disc displacement without reduction and various degrees of OA. They used a multiple logistic regression analysis and reported a significant increase in risk for an unsuccessful outcome in patients with a pretreatment report of chronic TMJ pain. Finally, Gu et al [42] reported on the effect of intra-articular irrigation injection therapy on OA of the TMJ. They treated 37 patients (the test group) with an intra-articular irrigation (arthrocentesis) and 26 with an intra-articular injection of steroid only. The percentages of patients rated as excellent or good in the two groups were 86% (arthrocentesis group) and 65% (steroid group), and the authors claimed this difference was statistically significant.

One possible reason why arthrocentesis is seldom used in the elderly is that their OA of the TMJ appears to be self-limiting, results in mild-to-moderate dysfunction, and is usually managed well with traditional nonsurgical therapy. The data discussed previously suggest that arthrocentesis-based lavage of the TMJ can be effective in increasing range of motion and decreasing pain in cases not responding to medical management, but that it should be restricted to cases with recent-onset hypomobility.

Polyjoint osteoarthritis and the temporomandibular joint in the elderly

Polyjoint or generalized OA is generally classified as either primary or secondary. The most common sign of a primary polyjoint OA is when the patient demonstrates the formation of Heberden's nodes on his or her distal interphalangeal joint of the hand. The proximal interphalangeal joint, the first carpometacarpal joint, and the spine, knee, and hip joints are also common OA sites. Primary polyjoint OA is more or less considered idiopathic, although genetic defects are suspected strongly in this disease, especially when a familial pattern of OA is present [22,26,43,44]. Secondary polyjoint OA is defined as joint damage or cartilage changes characteristic of OA caused by other disorders [43,45]. Secondary polyjoint OA may present in congenital and developmental disorders. Prior trauma, surgery, inflammatory disease, bone disease, blood dyscrasias, neuropathic joint diseases, excessively frequent intra-articular steroid injections, endocrinopathies, and metabolic disorders may damage joint surfaces and cartilage [22,44,45]. Finally, in cases of severe and aggressive polyjoint OA, a negative serologic test for rheumatoid factors should be obtained before the diagnosis of polyjoint or generalized OA is made.

The genetic defects most likely to be discovered involve the type-2 cartilage collagen binding proteins. This molecule forms a three-dimensional cross-linked fiber network with proteoglycan, creating compressibility and elasticity of the joint surface [22]. In addition to overt genetic defects, aging appears to decrease the ability of articular cartilage to withstand loading pressures and thus to promote cartilage degradation. In a recent review, Jordan et al [46] state that a formal study of the genetics of OA has only recently been undertaken. They discuss the findings from twin studies, segregation analyses, linkage analyses, and candidate gene association studies and summarize important information about inheritance patterns and the location of potentially causative mutations in the genome. Unfortunately, the various studies have not always agreed on the genetic factors to blame. This discordance probably results from variations in study populations, disease definitions, evaluation of control subjects, and statistical analysis. Nevertheless, most genetic researchers interested in OA believe that a complex of genetic defects will be identified in the near future.

Rheumatic arthritis and the temporomandibular joint in the elderly

RA is a chronic, systemic, autoimmune inflammatory disorder that is characterized by joint inflammation, erosive properties, and symmetric multiple joint involvement. RA can involve other body organs and is an aggressive disease causing joint damage within 2 years, decreased function, and increased impairment. It shortens life spans by 5 to 7 years [47–49] and, if severe, significantly alters the quality of life. The main serologic marker, rheumatoid factor (RF), an IgM autoantibody against constant fragment portion of an IgG molecule, is found in 75% to 80% of patients. Although the cause is unknown, certain genetic markers, namely HLA-DR4 and DR1, are found in approximately 30% of patients with RA. Familial studies offer strong evidence for genetic factors. Some evidence suggests that an infectious agent (eg, virus, bacteria) may trigger the disease in genetically predisposed individuals. Edema, hyperplasia of synovial lining, and inflammatory infiltrate are early components of RA onset. Chronic RA is characterized by hyperplasia of type-A synovial cells and subintimal mononuclear cell infiltration, resulting in massive damage to cartilage, bone, and tendons by the pannus, an infiltrating inflammatory synovial tissue mass [47–50].

Although RA is found in the TMJ, it appears to be one of the last joints attacked by RA. The TMJ is affected in more than 50% of adults and children with RA [51]. Clinical findings include dull aching pain associated with function, joint edema, and limited mandibular range of motion. Anterior open bites are common. Morning stiffness or stiffness at rest lasting longer than 1 hour is common. Radiographic findings range from flattening of the condylar head to severe, irregular deformity. Multiple joints are typically involved. Symmetric polyarthritis of at least three joints in 14 areas is found in 50% of patients. Laboratory tests for serum RF are positive [47,51].

Pharmacologic treatment of localized or polyjoint arthritis affecting the temporomandibular joint

Pharmacologic treatment of all types of arthritis includes nonnarcotic oral analgesics, such as acetaminophen, in patients with pain complaints. When NSAIDs are used, efficacy, cost, adverse reactions, and comorbidity should be considered; complications of peptic ulcer and bleeding can be serious in the geriatric patient. Renal function should be monitored. Cyclooxygenase–2 (COX-2) inhibitor NSAIDs, such as Celecoxib, cause less gastrointestinal injury because they selectively inhibit the isoenzyme COX-2. They also have a reduced effect on platelet aggregation and bleeding time.

Acetic acids (eg, Sulindac) are said to have a lower rate of renal adverse reactions than other NSAIDs. Indomethicin is poorly tolerated by the geriatric patient. Ibuprofen and naproxen, propionic acids, may be useful. Piroxicam can be taken once a day. Salicylates are less useful in the elderly because of gastrointestinal and central nervous system effects. Salsalate, a nonacetylated salicylate, does not affect platelet function and has minimal gastrointestinal toxicity. Oral corticosteroids have little use in the treatment of OA [51,52], but intra-articular corticosteroid injections may be useful in inflamed joints.

For the more aggressive RA cases that medications such as NSAIDs are not strong enough to manage, the current standard is to use one or more disease-modifying antirheumatic drugs (DMARDs) and a short course of oral or intra-articular steroid. DMARDs act slowly over 1 to 3 months. They appear to alter RA by causing erosive healing, controlling in-flammation, and improving function. In practice, the effectiveness of DMARDs varies by patient. DMARDs include antimalarial drug, sulfazalazine, intramuscular gold, methotrexate, hydroxychloroquine, cy-closporine, azathioprine, leflunomide, and cyclophosphamide. Treatment goals in RA include control of immunologic and inflammatory disease pro-cess, prevention of joint damage, normalization of function and life span, complete relief of symptoms, return to normal daily activities, avoidance of complications of the disease and its treatments, education, counseling, and physical and occupational therapy [47,52].

Development of new and combined medication regimens is leading to better management. Unique and progressive regimens, such as the use of tumor necrosis factor alpha antagonists in refractory RA, are giving hope to patients with severe disease. Recent work by Alhadaq and Moa [53] with tissue engineering is providing an exciting look into the future. These researchers harvested three tissue-engineered TMJ condyles from host mice. The harvested condyles formed from adult stem cells stimulated to form either bow or cartilage. Although this is early research, someday it may be possible to grow "new" condyles to replace diseased ones.

When they understand the influence of genetics, function, and trauma in the initiation of rheumatoid disorders, practitioners can establish clear, reasonable, and attainable treatment goals. We must take time to empower our patients to manage their disease through education, understanding, and reasonable expectations.

Summary and recommendations

The preponderance of data on TMJ is based on patients between the ages of 20 and 50. Very few studies have examined the efficacy of treatment methods for monoarticular or polyarticular disease involving the TMJ. With this caveat, the author offers the following conclusions and recommenda-tions based on the available literature and his own clinical experience:

Conclusions

In most studies where multimodal physical medicine therapy (eg, occlusal appliances, exercises, short-term use of NSAIDs, plus heat/ice and general advice about reduced jaw function) was used, this method produced a positive response in approximately 75% of patients.

The aforementioned treatment approach does not cure the derangement or arthritis; at present, this is not possible.

Judicious use of corticosteroid injections into the superior joint space of the painful TMJ is also a safe and logical therapy for many patients, with a low risk of morbidity and a high likelihood of symptom reduction.

In some patients, this approach will not be adequate, but the percentage of patients who state that they require further treatment is approximately 2%.

When the symptoms linger and do not respond to the above methods, it is likely that some causative factor is still present (eg, strong bruxism or tooth clenching habit, a generalized stress reaction, or an autoimmune disease process).

Therapeutic recommendations

For the patient with all forms of TMJ pain or disk–condyle incoordination (clicking), joint noises are usually managed with strict click avoidance instructions and hinge exercises. This self-directed treatment has the potential to stop and slow the progression of a dysfunctional clicking joint. A new and potentially viable therapy for the most noxious, disturbing joint clicks is the infusion of 1 mL of hyaluronan into the joint space as a method of reducing friction and promoting healing adaptation. This infusion can be performed up to four times (every 3 weeks) in a 1-year period.

For the patient with recent-onset TMJ closed locking, both manual manipulation (with or without anesthetic block of the TMJ) and arthrocentesis-assisted manipulation are logical first-line methods to manage most of the acute cases. Following the manipulation, the physician should institute a series of passive-stretching sessions of the jaw closers.

Open locking of the TMJ is largely avoidable with proper instruction once the locking has been manually reduced. For the patient with recurrent TMJ open locking, a series of hyaluronan injections is the first line of therapy; the second is referral to an oral surgeon for consideration of an arthroscopic surgery to stretch the joint capsule ligament structures or remove the bony abnormality that is inducing the locking.

For TMJ pain due to a polyarthritic diseases process (eg, RA) more specific disease-modifying drugs (eg, immunosuppressive medications) are in order.

The use of occlusal appliances for TMJ pain is indicated in the patient with a clear-cut jaw-muscle clenching or grinding behavior or an unstable occlusion.

Regarding efficacy, it should be noted that most of the individual modalities and methods described here have not been tested in randomized, controlled clinical trials on the specific TMJ disorder with which they appear logically matched. However, multiple clinical case series experiments show that the success rate for physical medicine methods in the management of unspecified TMJ disorder patients is around 75%, depending on the definition of success.

References

[1] Lawrence RC, Helmick CG, Arnett FC, et al. Estimates of the prevalence of arthritis and selected musculoskeletal disorders in the United States. Arthritis Rheum 1998;41:778–99.
[2] Felson DT. An update on the pathogenesis and epidemiology of osteoarthritis. Radiol Clin North Am 2004;42(1):1–9, v.
[3] Felson DT, Lawrence RC, Dieppe PA, et al. Osteoarthritis: new insights. Part 1: The disease and its risk factors. Ann Intern Med 2000;133(8):635–46.
[4] National Institute of Arthritis and Musculoskeletal and Skin Diseases. Arthritis prevalence rising as baby boomers grow older. 1998 NIH Press Release. Available at: www.niams.nih.gov/ne/press/1998/05_05.htm. Accessed June 2004.
[5] Lobbezzo-Scholte AM, De Leeuw JR, Steenks MH, et al. Diagnostic subgroups of craniomandibular disorders. Part I: Self-report data and clinical findings. J Orofac Pain 1995;9:24–36.
[6] Arthritis Foundation. The facts about arthritis. Available at: www.arthritis.org/resources/gettingstarted/default.asp. Accessed June 2004.
[7] Rugh JD, Solberg WK. Oral health status in the United States. Temporomandibular disorders. J Dent Educ 1985;49:389–404.
[8] Schiffman E, Fricton JR. Epidemiology of TMJ and craniofacial pain. In: Fricton JR, Kroening RJ, Hathaway KM, editors. TMJ and craniofacial pain: diagnosis and management. St. Louis (MO): Ishiaku Euro American; 1988. p. 1–10.
[9] DeKanter RJAM, Truin GJ, Burgersdijk RCW, et al. Prevalence in the Dutch adult population and a meta-analysis of signs and symptoms of temporomandibular disorders. J Dent Res 1993;72:1509–18.
[10] Dworkin SF, Huggins KH, Le Resche L, et al. Epidemiology of signs and symptoms in temporomandibular disorders: clinical signs in cases and controls. J Am Dent Assoc 1990; 120:273–81.
[11] Huber NU, Hall EH. A comparison of the signs of temporomandibular dysfunction and occlusal discrepancies in symptom free populations of men and women. Oral Surg Oral Med Oral Pathol 1990;70:180–3.
[12] Matsuka Y, Yatani H, Kuboki T, et al. Temporomandibular disorders in the adult population of Okayama City, Japan. Cranio 1996;14(2):158–62.
[13] Widmalm SE, Westesson PL, Kim IK, et al. Temporomandibular joint pathology related to age, sex, and dentition in autopsy material. Oral Surg Oral Med Oral Pathol 1994;78:416–25.
[14] Peirera FJ Jr, Lundh H, Westesson PL. Morphologic changes in the temporomandibular joint in different age groups: an autopsy investigation. Oral Surg Oral Med Oral Pathol 1994; 78:279–87.
[15] Bell WE. Temporomandibular disorders: classification, diagnosis, management. 3rd edition. Chicago: Year Book Medical Publishers; 1990.

[16] Boering G. Temporomandibular joint osteoarthritis: an analysis of 400 cases—a clinical and radiographic investigation [thesis]. Groningen (Netherlands): Department of Oral and Maxillofacial Surgery, University of Groningen; 1966 [reprinted 1994].

[17] De Leeuw R, Boering G, Stegenga B, et al. Symptoms of temporomandibular joint osteoarthritis and internal derangement 30 years after non-surgical treatment. J Craniomandibular Pract 1995;13:81–8.

[18] Kaminishi R. Metabolic factors of the TMJ. In: McNeill C., editor. Current controversies in temporomandibular joint disorders. Proceedings of the Craniomandibular Institute's 10th Annual Squaw Valley Winter Seminar. Chicago(IL): Quintessence Publishing; 1991. p. 57–9.

[19] Byers PD, Maroudas A, Oztop F, et al. Histological and biochemical studies on cartilage from osteoarthrotic femoral heads with special reference to surface characteristics. Connect Tissue Res 1977;5:41–9.

[20] Mankin HJ, Thrassher AZ. Water content and binding in normal and osteoarthritic human cartilage. J Bone Joint Surg 1975;557(A):76–80.

[21] Blaustein DI, Scapino RP. Remodeling of the TMJ disc and posterior attachment in disc displacement specimens in relation to glycosaminoglycan content. Plast Reconstr Surg 1986; 78:756–64.

[22] Sah RL, Chen AC, Chen SS, et al. Articular cartilage repair. In: Koopman W, editor. Arthritis and allied conditions—a textbook of rheumatology. Philadelphia: Lippincott Williams & Wilkins; 2001. p. 2264–73.

[23] Nannmark U, Sennerby L, Haraldson T. Macroscopic, microscopic and radiologic assessment of the condylar part of the TMJ in elderly subjects. An autopsy study. Swed Dent J 1990;14(4):163–9.

[24] Nakayama Y, Narita T, Mori A, et al. The effects of age and sex on chondroitin sulfates in normal synovial fluid. Arthritis Rheum 2002;46(8):2105–8.

[25] DeGroot J, Verzijl N, Wenting-Van Wijk MJ, et al. Age-related decrease in susceptibility of human articular cartilage to matrix metalloproteinase–mediated degradation: the role of advanced glycation end products. Arthritis Rheum 2001;44(11):2562–71.

[26] Felson DT, Lawrence RC, Dieppe PA, et al. Osteoarthritis: new insights. Part 2: The disease and its risk factors. Ann Intern Med 2000;133(9):726–37.

[27] Dulcic N, Panduric J, Kraljevic S, et al. Frequency of internal derangement of the temporomandibular joint in elderly individuals. Eur J Med Res 2003;8(10):465–71.

[28] Gillette JA, Tarricone R. Economic evaluation of osteoarthritis treatment in Europe. Expert Opin Pharmacother 2003;4(3):327–41.

[29] Hiltunen K, Vehkalahti MM, Peltola JS, et al. A 5-year follow-up of occlusal status and radiographic findings in mandibular condyles of the elderly. Int J Prosthodont 2002;15(6): 539–43.

[30] Kopp S, Carlsson GE, Haraldson T, et al. Long-term effect of intra-articular injections of sodium hyaluronate and corticosteroid on temporomandibular joint arthritis. J Oral Maxillofac Surg 1987;45(11):929–35.

[31] Alstergren P, Appelgren A, Appelgren B, et al. The effect on joint fluid concentration of neuropeptide Y by intra-articular injection of glucocorticoid in temporomandibular joint arthritis. Acta Odontol Scand 1996;54(1):1–7.

[32] Vallon D, Akerman S, Nilner M, et al. Long-term follow-up of intra-articular injections into the temporomandibular joint in patients with rheumatoid arthritis. Swed Dent J 2002;26(4): 149–58.

[33] Huskisson EC, Donnelly S. Hyaluronic acid in the treatment of osteoarthritis of the knee. Rheumatology (Oxford) 1999;38(7):602–7.

[34] Wen DY. Intra-articular hyaluronic acid injections for knee osteoarthritis. Am Fam Physician 2000;62:565–70, 572.

[35] Bertolami CN, Gay T, Clark GT, et al. Use of sodium hyaluronate in treating temporomandibular joint disorders: a randomized, double-blind, placebo-controlled clinical trial. J Oral Maxillofac Surg 1993;51(3):232–42.

[36] Shi ZD, Yang F, Zhang JY, et al. [Randomized controlled trial of sodium hyaluronate for degenerative disorders of the temporomandibular joint.] Zhongguo Xiu Fu Chong Jian Wai Ke Za Zhi 2002;16(1):11–5 [in Chinese].

[37] Winocur E, Gavish A, Halachmi M, et al. Topical application of capsaicin for the treatment of localized pain in the temporomandibular joint area. J Orofac Pain 2000;14(1):31–6.

[38] Myrer JW, Feland JB, Fellingham GW. The effects of a topical analgesic and placebo in treatment of chronic knee pain. J Aging Phys Act 2004;12(2):199–213.

[39] Burch F, Codding C, Patel N, et al. Lidocaine patch 5% improves pain, stiffness, and physical function in osteoarthritis pain patients: a prospective, multicenter, open-label effectiveness trial. Osteoarthritis Cartilage 2004;12(3):253–5.

[40] Nitzan DW, Price A. The use of arthrocentesis for the treatment of osteoarthritic temporomandibular joints. J Oral Maxillofac Surg 2001;59(10):1154–9 [discussion: 1160].

[41] Emshoff R, Rudisch A. Determining predictor variables for treatment outcomes of arthrocentesis and hydraulic distention of the temporomandibular joint. J Oral Maxillofac Surg 2004;62(7):816–23.

[42] Gu ZY, Wu HL, Wu QL, et al. The effect of intra-articular irrigation injection therapy on osteoarthrosis of the temporomandibular joint. Chin J Dent Res 1998;1(3):44–8.

[43] Malemud CJ, Islam N, Haqqi M. Pathophysiological mechanisms in osteoarthritis lead to novel therapeutic strategies. Cells Tissues Organs 2003;174(1–2):34–48.

[44] Lozada C, Altman RD. Management of osteoarthritis. In: Koopman W, editor. Arthritis and allied conditions—a textbook of rheumatology. Philadelphia: Lippincott Williams & Wilkins; 2001. p. 2246–58.

[45] Beary JF, Luggen ME. Osteoarthritis. In: Paget SA, Gibofsky A, Beary JF, editors. Manual of rheumatological and outpatient orthopedic disorders. 4th edition. Philadelphia: Lippincott Williams & Wilkins; 2000. p. 337–48.

[46] Jordan JM, Kraus VB, Hochberg MC. Genetics of osteoarthritis. Curr Rheumatol Rep 2004;6(1):7–13.

[47] Mevorach D, Paget SA. Rheumatoid arthritis. In: Paget SA, Gibofsky A, Beary JF, editors. Manual of rheumatological and outpatient orthopedic disorders. 4th edition. Philadelphia: Lippincott Williams & Wilkins; 2000. p. 193–228.

[48] Fox DA. Etiology and pathogenesis of rheumatoid arthritis. In: Koopman W, editor. Arthritis and allied conditions—a textbook of rheumatology. Philadelphia: Lippincott Williams & Wilkins; 2001. p. 55.

[49] Hale LP, Haynes BF. Pathology of rheumatoid arthritis and associated disorders. In: Koopman W, editor. Arthritis and allied conditions—a textbook of rheumatology. Philadelphia: Lippincott Williams & Wilkins; 2001. p. 56.

[50] Jasin H. Mechanisms of tissue damage in rheumatoid arthritis. In: Koopman W, editor. Arthritis and allied conditions—a textbook of rheumatology. Philadelphia: Lippincott Williams & Wilkins; 2001. p. 57.

[51] Dolwick FM. Temporomandibular disorders. In: Koopman W, editor. Arthritis and allied conditions—a textbook of rheumatology. Philadelphia: Lippincott Williams & Wilkins; 2001. p. 2019–25.

[52] Furst DE, Hillson J. Therapeutic approaches in the rheumatic diseases. In: Koopman W, editor. Arthritis and allied conditions—a textbook of rheumatology. Philadelphia: Lippincott Williams & Wilkins; 2001. p. 671–703.

[53] Alhadaq A, Mao JJ. Tissue-engineered neogenesis of human-shaped mandibular condyle from rat mesenchymal stem cells. Dent Res 2003;82(12):951–6.

THE DENTAL
CLINICS
OF NORTH AMERICA

Dent Clin N Am 49 (2005) 343–362

Orofacial Pain and Sensory Disorders in the Elderly

Glenn T. Clark, DDS, MS*, Hajime Minakuchi, DDS, PhD, Ana C. Lotaif, DDS, MS

Division of Diagnostic Sciences, University of Southern California, School of Dentistry, 925 West 34th Street, Room B-14, Los Angeles, CA 90089-0641, USA

An elderly patient who attends his or her physician's or dentist's office with a complaint of pain is more likely to be taking multiple medications and to have two or more active chronic medical problems than is a patient 2 or 3 decades younger. Likewise, the diagnostic process and time needed to investigate the pain complaint will be more complex for the older patient. The prevalence of general pain in the elderly population is moderately high, with estimates of persistent pain ranging from 25% to 88%, depending on the definition used and the nature of the population [1,2]. Chronic pain is defined as pain that persists beyond the time expected for healing. Alternatively, chronic pain may be due to a long-standing persistent disease process, such as an autoimmune disease or neurologic sensitization in peripheral or central nerves. In the elderly, the cause of chronic pain is frequently neuropathy or polyarthritis. Riley et al [3] conducted telephone interviews of community-dwelling older (≥65) north Floridians (N = 1636) and found that 17.4% reported some form of current or recent (ie, within the last year) orofacial pain. The pains were generally of four types: jaw joint pain, facial pain, burning mouth pain, and oral sores. In this article the authors discuss the likely disorders and diseases that produce facial pain and burning pain in the mouth. They do not cover jaw joint pain, oral sores, or ulceration-induced pain, as these conditions are better discussed in the context of arthritis and oral pathologies of the mouth. At the same time, the authors supplement their discussion with that of another disease category seen in the elderly, namely, occlusal dysesthesia.

---

* Corresponding author.
E-mail address: gtc@usc.edu (G.T. Clark).

0011-8532/05/$ - see front matter © 2005 Elsevier Inc. All rights reserved.
doi:10.1016/j.cden.2004.10.011   *dental.theclinics.com*

Facial pain related to oral motor disorders

An oral motor disorder is a "movement disorder," and they can be broadly classified into "hypokinetic" and "hyperkinetic" conditions. The hypokinetic disorders (eg, parkinsonian rigidity) are not associated with pain. By contrast, the hyperkinesias can and do produce pain. These can be subclassified into the stereotypic dyskinesias, tremors, dystonias, tics, myoclonus, and choreas. Some might even add the parasomnias (eg, sleep bruxism, periodic leg movement syndrome) and secondary spasms to this group. All movement disorders, and oral movement disorders in particular, are more common in older age. Bourgeois et al [4] examined 270 elderly subjects in a residential nursing facility for dyskinesias, both spontaneous and drug-induced. They reported that females were twice as likely to have a dyskinesia (27%) as males (12%). Among those who had dyskinesia, two thirds of the dyskinesias were related to neuroleptic medications and one third were of spontaneous onset. The good news is that, although some oral motor disorders do induce pain, the link between pain and abnormal motor function is generally not strong. The hyperkinetic disorders that produce pain are discussed later.

Dystonia presents as an involuntary, briefly sustained contraction of muscles. If the dystonic contraction is strong and frequent enough, pain may result. When the dystonia involves only one or two areas of the body, it is labeled a focal dystonia. For example, some patients exhibit an involuntary repetitive contraction of the orbicularis oculi muscles, which produce eye closure. This disorder has been called blepharospasm. If the cervical (usually sternocleidomastoid and trapezius muscles) contract, this is called a torticollis. Several focal dystonic patterns involving some combination of jaw, neck, tongue, and perioral muscles are described as focal orofacial, orolingual, oromandibular, or cervical dystonias [5]. Frequently, the patient with a significant oromandibular dystonia will have compromised mastication and be unable to function with a removable dental prosthesis (especially mandibular full dentures). Some of the severe orofacial dystonias may actually create such difficulty that patients are unable to eat and lose weight. If the dystonia strongly affects the tongue musculature, it may compromise the patient's ability to speak clearly. A combination of blepharospasm and jaw opening dystonia has been labeled Meige's syndrome [6,7].

Bruxism is another example of a frequently seen motor disorder that, if severe, produces pain and even damage to the masticatory structures, such as broken or worn teeth, derangement, temporomandibular joint (TMJ) arthritis, and jaw muscle pain. Between 6% and 20% of the population have been reported to exhibit bruxism. This disorder is more common in children (14%) and generally decreases after the age of 50 years [8]. The distinction between tooth grinding and tooth clenching is not clear-cut, but the latter is thought to occur more frequently and to be more common in women than in men. Actually, it is somewhat difficult to confirm or refute the presence of bruxism or clenching, because patients often do not know they are grinding and certainly may not know they are clenching. Moreover, there has been no population-based study involving large numbers of patients in which polysomnography has been performed. Dental wear or attrition is not always a good indicator of current bruxism or clenching.

The causation is not clear for any of the spontaneous-onset motor disorders, whether one is discussing dystonia or bruxism. A causative agent can be identified when the movement disorder is secondary to a prescription medication or abuse drug [9]. The most commonly reported offending drug regimen is chronic exposure to neuroleptic drugs. A wide range of other drugs have been linked to involuntary movements, usually by isolated case reports in the literature, although it is often difficult to evaluate the clinical significance of such reports. One class of medications recently associated with motor side effects is the serotonin selective reuptake inhibitors (eg, paroxetine, fluoxitine). Winocur et al [10] reviewed the literature on drug-induced bruxism and concluded that, despite the widespread anecdotal case reports, there is insufficient evidence-based data to draw definite conclusions about the effects of various drugs on bruxism. Although certain substances related to the dopaminergic, serotonergic, and adrenergic systems suppress or exacerbate bruxist activity in humans and animals, the literature is still controversial. Evaluation of a patient's drug history may prevent oral motor dysfunction or identify an iatrogenic cause.

Oral motor dysfunction is best managed with a multidisciplinary approach, including medications, protective devices (bite guards), and motor-paralyzing injections (ie, botulinum toxin). The protocol for these injections has been described in a recent review [11]. One common medication used in this disorder is high-dose anticholinergic medication (trihexyphenidyl); however, older patients tolerate this drug poorly, and it works in only one third of those to whom it is prescribed. Side effects consist of substantial dryness of the mouth, jitteriness, stomatitis, blurred vision, and forgetfulness.

Facial pain related to muscle pain (myalgia, myofascial pain, and fibromyalgia)

Localized myalgia, regional myofascial pain, and the more generalized fibromyalgia syndrome (FMS) are common chronic pain problems that predominantly affect middle-aged women [12]. Although local myalgia and myofascial pain are more prevalent in the middle aged, fibromyalgia increases with age and is substantially more evident in the elderly population. FMS affects up to 2% of the population and can start at any age; it is at least seven times more common in women than in men [13]. By the time the diagnosis is made, patients have often had symptoms for many years. Patients with fibromyalgia complain of pervasive muscular and sometimes joint pain and, by definition, have pain on both sides of the body, above and below the waist and in both the trunk and the extremities. These findings suggest (and most researchers agree) that an aberrant central pain processing mechanism produces a state of sensitized pain perception in FMS [14]. Because of the widespread muscle and joint pain, fibromyalgia patients usually have poor quality, nonrestorative sleep. They also frequently report irritable bowel syndrome and headaches. Because of the negative effect fibromyalgia has on activities of daily living, it usually induces depression and anxiety, and it often accompanies other chronic, painful disorders [15]. Specific clinical history and examination criteria must be met before a diagnosis of fibromyalgia is given. These criteria, adopted by the American College of Rheumatology [16], specify that a diagnosis of fibromyalgia is made when the patient has widespread pain for at least 3 months accompanied by tenderness at discrete locations. To be eligible for research studies, patients must have at least 11 tender points out of a possible 18, but, in practice, the diagnosis can be made in patients with fewer tender points if there is widespread pain and many of the other characteristic symptoms. Patients with fibromyalgia often are tender all over; the presence of tenderness in locations other than the classic ones does not exclude the diagnosis.

Medications often used for FMS are listed in Table 1. The most common medication used in this group of patients is a tricyclic antidepressant agent (eg, nortriptyline, amitriptyline) [17]. These medications are versatile and effective in treating many symptoms associated with FMS, but tolerability remains a problem, and this is especially true in the elderly. By contrast, serotonin selective reuptake inhibitors show improved tolerability and have demonstrated much clearer activity against depressed mood in the context of FMS than have tricyclic antidepressants. However, their activity against other symptoms appears less robust. Sedative-hypnotic compounds, such as zolpidem (Ambien) appear to be useful adjuncts for the treatment of disturbed sleep, and the use of tramadol to treat FMS pain is supported by three trials. Nonsteroidal anti-inflammatory drugs, by contrast, have not been shown to be particularly effective in FMS.

Table 1
Medications for myofascial pain and fibromyalgia

Medication class	Effect	Comments
Tricyclic anti-depressant agents (eg, nortriptyline)	+++	Moderately to mildly helpful for pain, but high side effects
Serotonin selective reuptake inhibitors (eg, citalopram)	+	Lower side effects than TCAs; more for depression than for pain
Opioid/SNRI: serotonin-norepinephrine reuptake inhibitor/narcotic (eg, tramadol)	+++	Several studies show it is moderately helpful for FMS-related pain.
NSAIDs (eg, ibuprofen)	+/−	Not particularly effective in FMS

Abbreviations: NSAIDs, nonsteroidal anti-inflammatory drugs; TCAs, tricyclic anti-depressants.

Behavioral treatments entail making sure the patient has a good understanding of the disorder and engages in daily physical exercise and relaxation. The self-management program is crucial to ensuring that the patient does not have increasing feelings of anxiety and helplessness, which aggravate the disease [18]. Many patients can be helped by encouragement and reassurance, along with regular aerobic exercise. However, patients with fibromyalgia tend to remain symptomatic at unchanged levels for many years. Most, if not all, should be encouraged to continue working and to maintain regular social activities despite their symptoms. The management of fibromyalgia patients involves a complex interplay between pharmaco-logic management of pain and associated symptoms and nonpharmacologic modalities. Regular follow-up and modification of the initial management strategy is usually required, depending on the response pattern. FMS patients typically have a number of complaints beyond pain, and a vast majority cite fatigue as a significant cause of morbidity. The potential causes of fatigue in these patients are manifold, but recent evidence suggests that sleep disturbances play a particularly important role. Exercise interventions for these patients vary, depending on the extent and severity of symptoms as well as on factors that affect patient motivation and adherence. Secondary psychosocial effects are pervasive, including depression, reduced confidence in one's ability to manage the disease, and disruption of relationships with friends and family. Unfortunately, depression and reduced self-confidence make it particularly difficult for these patients to adhere to an exercise program.

Facial pain of vascular origin

Facial pain can result from a generalized chronic vascular inflammatory syndrome of large and middle-sized blood vessels that is characterized by the presence of giant cell accumulation inside the arteries. When giant cell arteritis predominantly affects the cranial and scalp vessels, it is called temporal arteritis, and the palpable vessels of the scalp are usually sore, tender, thickened, and pulseless [19]. Temporal arteritis commonly presents for the first time in older people; the mean age at onset is 70 years, with most cases occurring between 60 and 75 years. It is rare in people less than 50 years of age [20]. Women are affected twice as often as men. Temporal arteritis is probably a polygenic disease in which multiple environmental and genetic factors influence susceptibility and severity. Genetic polymorphisms have also been considered important candidates for factors of susceptibility to giant cell arteritis and polymyalgia rheumatica, a similar disorder. However, additional studies are required to clarify the genetic influence on susceptibility to these conditions.

Gonzalez-Gay et al [21] examined the influence of age on the clinical expression of giant cell arteritis in a population in northwest Spain. Using patients with biopsy-proven giant cell arteritis, they reported that this disorder was more common in women (rate ratio 1.58 [females] to 1.00 [males]) and occurred in patients with an age greater than or equal to 50 years. Systemic symptoms (eg, fever) occur in about half of patients; in approximately 15% of patients, this may be the presenting clinical manifestation. In approximately two thirds of patients, headache is the most frequent presenting symptom. The onset tends to be gradual but can also be abrupt, with new headache pain, such as scalp tenderness, as a primary complaint. The pain symptoms are usually confined to the temporal and sometimes the occipital arteries, but the occipital arteries are less often involved. Intermittent claudication (fatigue or pain on function) may occur in the muscles of the jaw or even tongue. In rare cases, more marked vascular narrowing may lead to infarction of the scalp or the tongue. One serious complication of temporal arteritis is permanent partial or complete loss of vision in one or both eyes. Affected patients typically report partially obscured vision in one eye, which may progress to total blindness. If untreated, the other eye is likely to become affected within 1 to 2 weeks. Warning signals for temporal arteritis include onset of a new headache after the age of 50 and the progressive course and systemic symptoms of malaise and jaw claudication on function. The screening investigations usually ordered for clinically suspected temporal arteritis are complete blood count, erythrocyte sedimentation rate (ESR), C reactive protein, urea electrolytes, liver function, glucose, thyroid function, rheumatoid factor, electrophoresis, and chest radiography. If the ESR is elevated, a biopsy of a clinically affected scalp vessel should immediately be performed; if there is no clearly involved vessel, the superficial temporal artery ipsilateral to the headache should be sampled. If the clinical situation suggests giant cell arteritis, a biopsy should be performed even if the ESR is not elevated, because the disease is sometimes found on biopsy in patients without ESR elevation [22].

Temporal arteritis is usually treated with corticosteroids in a dose sufficient to relieve symptoms and normalize the ESR [23]. A usual starting regimen is 80 mg of prednisone daily. The dose of steroid may be regarded as balancing the risk for relapse and complications of the disease process against the risk for steroid-induced side effects. It is important to adhere to the correct dosage and regimen of steroid treatment to avoid both undertreatment (resulting in increased risk for arteritic complications) and overtreatment (resulting in increased risk for steroid-associated side effects). The National Osteoporosis Guidelines (http://www.rcplondon.ac.uk/pubs/wp_osteo_update.htm) state that individuals on more than 7.5 mg of prednisolone for more than 6 months should be given osteoporosis prophylaxis. Calcium and vitamin D supplementation should be given with corticosteroid therapy in all patients with temporal arteritis. The treatment for temporal arteritis can be divided in four parts. Part 1: the starting dose of 20 to 40 mg prednisolone can be maintained for 1 month but should be supplemented with an osteoporosis prophylaxis medication. Part 2: once the clinical symptoms have been reduced, the dose of prednisolone can be reduced by 5 mg every 2 weeks. Once a daily dose of 5 mg per day is achieved, it is wise to hold the patient at this daily dose for 12 months. If there is no recurrence, this dosage can be stopped.

Facial pain of neurovascular origin

Approximately 66% of headache pain in the elderly is caused by migraines or tension-type headaches, and this figure is well over 90% in a younger cohort [24]. Unfortunately, when new headaches develop in the elderly, the other 33% are more likely to be due to an intracranial lesion or a systemic disease. The good news is that the overall prevalence of headaches declines with age; indeed, this prevalence has been reported to decline from 83% in individuals between 21 and 34 years to 59% in those between ages 55 and 74 [25]. One exception to this pattern is that migraines sometimes occur for the first time after age 50; about 2% of all migraines start at this late age [26].

It is prudent to diagnose systemic and intracranial diseases and other disorders that are often a cause of headaches in old age using CT or MRI of the head, just in case. Wilkinson [27] has described how auras tend to disappear with age, but one concern in the elderly is that transient ischemic attack might be mistaken as an aura and vice versa. A good general rule is that an unusual initial presentation or a change in symptomatology (other than frequency or intensity) of migraine is a "red flag" that calls for consideration of imaging studies.

Managing headaches in older patients presents several challenges [28]. First, diagnosis is always difficult, because of the possibility that the pain is due to a central nervous system pathology or some other organic disease process. Second, treating the elderly with migraine abortive medications (triptans) requires extra caution, because of their reduced tolerance to medications and potential for increased contraindications due to concomitant disease (eg, coronary artery disease) or polypharmacy. Third, the use of prophylaxis for the chronic daily headache sufferer (eg, beta blockers, tricyclic antidepressants, calcium channel blockers) may cause unacceptable lethargy and confusion in the elderly. These medications are usually more sedating and more apt to result in kidney failure because of the decreased renal reserve in this age group.

Facial pain related to trigeminal neuralgia

Trigeminal neuralgia (TN) presents as a sudden, usually unilateral, severe, brief, stabbing, recurrent pain in the distribution of one or more branches of the fifth cranial nerve. Although recent evidence points to vascular injury (abrasion) of the trigeminal nerve root within the cranial vault, this alteration is not usually visible using current imaging modalities.

However, as many as 15% of patients may have an underlying cause, such as a benign or malignant tumor of the posterior fossa or multiple sclerosis [29]. Some patients have many features of TN, yet aspects of their history do not agree with the typical manifestations of the condition. Many patients attribute their pain to dental causes and will seek dental therapy as a first line of treatment. Because dental pain is extremely common, this is a valid assumption; however, it is important that dentists consider possible nondental causes of pain and not attempt complex and irreversible procedures. TN may also present exclusively intraorally, a manifestation that can be confusing for patients and clinicians. The International Headache Society has suggested criteria for the diagnosis of TN (Box 1) [30].

Most drugs used in the management of TN interfere with ion channels, in line with the assumption that pain in TN is primarily caused by spontaneous ectopic neuronal firing [31]. Some drugs may also inhibit noxious transmission by reducing glutamate release and by augmenting segmental gamma-aminobutyric acid inhibition. The effects of both the drugs whose efficacy has been evidenced in controlled trials and most of those being used on the basis of uncontrolled observations seem to be sound and consistent with the proposed pathophysiologic mechanisms in TN and the basic pharmacology of the drugs. The current evidence leaves no doubt that carbamazepine should be the first-line treatment for patients with TN. Dosing according to efficacy and side effects is clinically feasible; after dose

---

Box 1. International Headache Society criteria for trigeminal neuralgia

- Paroxysmal attacks of facial or frontal pain that last from a few seconds to <2 minutes
- Pain has at least four of the following characteristics:
  (a) Distribution along one or more divisions of the trigeminal nerve
  (b) Sudden, intense, sharp, superficial, stabbing, or burning in quality
  (c) Severe intensity
  (d) Precipitation from trigger areas or by certain daily activities, such as eating, talking, washing the face, or cleaning the teeth
  (e) The patient is entirely asymptomatic between paroxysms.
- No neurologic deficit
- Attacks are stereotyped in the individual patient
- Exclusion of other causes of facial pain by history, physical examination findings, and special investigation (when necessary)

titration, the patients should preferably be given slow-release formulations, so that diurnal variations in serum drug levels do not influence efficacy. Carbamazepine and oxcarbazepine are similar in terms of basic pharmacology and may be interchangeable; moreover, oxcarbazepine appears to be better tolerated. However, the efficacy of oxcarbazepine needs to be evidenced in controlled trials. In some countries, despite the lack of controlled clinical trials, oxcarbazepine is the first drug of choice. The choice of treatment will, of course, also depend on patient-related factors. Elderly patients are more prone to some central nervous system side effects of carbamazepine, and some of the other drugs may be preferable for them. Carbamazepine cannot be used in patients with cardiac conduction disturbances.

Facial pain related to a chronic trigeminal neuropathy

Over the years, many different terms have been used to describe patients with dental pain of unknown origin. The most common is "atypical odontalgia" [32–37]; once the tooth is extracted and the pain continues, the term "phantom tooth pain" is used [38–41]. Although the mechanism is debated, this is most likely a neuropathic pain process, which is defined by the International Association for the Study of Pain [42] as "pain initiated or caused by a primary lesion, or dysfunction in the nervous system." In a recent paper, Marbach [43] introduced some specific diagnostic criteria for what he termed "phantom tooth pain," based mainly on the clinical characteristics of the pain.

Currently, the most accepted theory regarding these pain phenomena is that trauma to the orofacial structures (eg, traumatic injury, periodontal surgery, pulp extirpation, endodontic therapy, apicoectomy, tooth extraction, implant insertion) or even minor trauma (eg, crown preparation, inferior alveolar nerve block) alters the neural continuity of the tissues, creating sensitization of the peripheral nociceptive nerves. This mechanism falls into the category of neuropathic pain, in that, after the wound has healed, the neural tissue is responsible for the pain and other related symptoms (paresthesia, dysesthesia). Of course, multiple mechanisms are involved in the pathogenesis of neuropathic pain. But the bottom line is that, following a nerve injury or regional inflammation, the afferent nociceptive fibers become sensitized, showing a lower activation threshold and sometimes developing spontaneous ectopic activity as a result of increased expression or redistribution of sodium channels on the axon. This sensitization could easily explain some clinical manifestations of oral neuropathic pain, such as the clear-cut mechanical or thermal allodynia and persistent spontaneous pain.

The diagnosis of chronic trigeminal neuropathy is essentially a clinical process. The most prominent and sometimes the only evident symptom is pain. It is commonly described as a continuous and spontaneous dull ache localized in a tooth or tooth region. The location may change to an edentulous area or entire parts of the maxilla or mandible. The pain also may be described as burning, sharp, or throbbing. It usually persists for months or years, being continuous and persistent but oscillating in intensity, with episodes when the pain is more acute and severe. For a diagnosis of trigeminal neuropathy to be made, other pathologies characterized by tooth pain need to be ruled out. Several have been listed: pulpal toothache, TN, myofascial pain, sinusitis, cracked tooth syndrome, and migrainous neuralgia. Probably the most difficult task is to distinguish between trigeminal neuropathy and toothache from pulpal origin. Five character-istics that are common in trigeminal neuropathy but not in pulpal toothache are listed in Box 2.

Once the diagnosis of trigeminal neuropathy has been made, appropriate treatment needs to be established, including avoidance of any further dental procedure that could aggravate the pain. Most medications used are formulated for the treatment of neuropathic pain and appear to be effective in most patients with trigeminal neuropathy [44]. In many of the articles reviewed, tricyclic antidepressants (TCAs) were prescribed with good results. The use of these medications is limited by the occurrence of side effects; TCAs cause dry mouth, weight gain, constipation, and urinary retention. They are contraindicated in patients with angle-closure glaucoma or high intraocular pressure and those taking other medications, such as monoamine oxidase inhibitors, central nervous system depressants (eg, alcohol, barbiturates, narcotics), anticholinergics, and sympathomimetics, because of drug-to-drug interactions. It is usually possible to avoid or minimize the side effects by adjusting the dose or switching to a different medication within the same category (eg, nortriptyline has less anticholin-ergic effect than amitriptyline and imipramine). The primary alternative to TCAs is the mild anticonvulsant gabapentin, or clonazepam. Opioid narcotic analgesics (eg, oxycodone, meperidine, controlled-release mor-phine, fentanyl, ketamine, methadone) have been tried, but they are usually only moderately effective for neuropathic pain and produce unacceptable

---

Box 2. Five clinical features of trigeminal neuropathy

Constant pain is experienced in the tooth with no obvious
  source of local pathology.
Local provocation of the tooth does not relate consistently to
  the pain. Hot, cold, or loading stimulation does not reliably
  affect the pain.
The toothache is unchanging over weeks or months, whereas
  pulpal pain tends to worsen or improve with time.
Repeated dental therapies fail to resolve the pain.
Response to local anesthesia is often equivocal.

side effects in the elderly. Injections of local anesthetics alone or in combination with corticosteroids (triamcinalone) can be repeated and have been found effective as a management tool for many patients. Sympathetic and parasympathetic nerve blocks, through the stellate ganglia or sphenopalatine ganglia, have been reported with similar results.

Finally, medications applied to the site of the pain sometimes give good results. Capsaicin at a concentration of 0.025% for 4 weeks, eventually associated with a topical anesthetic if the treatment is too painful, and eutectic mixture of lidocaine and prilocaine bases cream at the concentration of 5% may be helpful.

Facial pain related to postherpetic neuralgia

Herpes zoster strikes millions of older adults annually worldwide and disables a substantial number of them by means of postherpetic neuralgia. The incidence of herpes zoster increases sharply among patients aged 50 to 60 years and continues its upward course in the decades after 60 [45]. Herpes zoster is caused by renewed replication and spread of varicella-zoster virus in sensory ganglia and afferent peripheral nerves in the setting of age-related, disease-related, or drug-related decline in cellular immunity to varicella-zoster virus. When reactivated, the varicella-zoster virus over-whelms immune control and spreads in the affected ganglia and sensory nerves to the skin. As already mentioned, this event is more likely to occur in elderly people, partially because of age-related decline in specific cell-mediated immune responses to varicella-zoster virus. The disease begins with localized abnormal skin sensations, ranging from itching or tingling to severe pain, which precede the skin lesions by 1 to 5 days. Healing of the skin lesions occurs over a period of 2 to 4 weeks and often results in scarring and permanent changes in pigmentation. The cutaneous eruption is unilateral and does not cross the midline. Along with the rash, most patients experience a dermatomal pain syndrome caused by acute neuritis. The neuritis is described as burning, deep aching, tingling, itching, or stabbing pain and ranges from mild to severe. This pain continues after the rash has healed in as many as 60% to 70% of people aged over 60 years and develops into postherpetic neuralgia.

Postherpetic neuralgia is the most frequently feared complication of herpes zoster in the elderly [46]. The best-established risk factors for postherpetic neuralgia are older age, immunocompromised status, and greater severity of acute pain and rash during zoster. The patient with postherpetic neuralgia may experience constant pain (described as burning, aching, or throbbing), intermittent pain (described as stabbing or shooting), and stimulus-evoked pain, such as allodynia (described as tender). Furthermore, postherpetic neuralgia can impair the elderly patient's functional status by interfering with basic activities of daily life, such as dressing, bathing, and mobility, and instrumental activities of daily life, such as traveling, shopping, cooking, and housework. The appearance of herpes zoster is sufficiently distinctive that a clinical diagnosis is usually accurate. A direct immunofluorescence assay, when needed, is the best way (other than culture) to distinguish herpes simplex virus infections from varicella-zoster virus infections. Polymerase-chain-reaction techniques are useful for detecting varicella-zoster virus DNA in fluid and tissues [47,48].

No single treatment has proved effective for postherpetic neuralgia [49]. Combination therapy and a consultation with a pain-management specialist are often required. No one treatment is uniformly effective in elderly patients with the disease. Patients and clinicians have employed a large number of treatments for postherpetic neuralgia, but few have been carefully evaluated. Recent clinical trials indicate that topical lidocaine, gabapentin, opiates, TCAs, and intrathecal methylprednisolone can significantly reduce pain in patients with postherpetic neuralgia. Treatment of the disease is complex, often requiring a multifaceted approach. Clinical trials have shown that opioids, TCAs, and gabapentin reduce the severity or duration of postherpetic neuralgia, either as single agents or in combination. The adverse effects of these medications can be additive, especially in elderly patients. Topical application of lidocaine patches has been a major therapeutic advance for some patients. Although multiple studies have demonstrated that antiviral therapy alone reduces the duration of pain, antiviral drugs do not reliably prevent postherpetic neuralgia. Chronic neuropathic pain will develop in a subgroup of patients despite appropriate antiviral treatment.

Burning mouth symptoms (not related to hyposalivation)

Stomatopyrosis (commonly called burning mouth syndrome) and its variant glossopyrosis (burning tongue) are chronic pain syndromes that mainly affect middle-aged and elderly subjects. The sufferers are typically within an age range from 38 to 78 years [50]. Occurrence below the age of 30 is rare, and the female-to-male ratio is about 7:1. Most (90%) of the women with these symptoms are peri- or postmenopausal women. Burning sensation is the main complaint and is usually described as constant, gradually increasing throughout the day, or intermittent, without any reliable alleviating agents. Diagnosis of burning mouth syndrome (BMS) is one of exclusion, because, as in other neurosensory disorders, there are no measurable physical signs other than pain. More than two thirds of BMS patients report a bitter, metallic taste sensation along with the burning. The BMS patient typically reports pain onset ranging from 3 years before to 12 years after menopause; approximately 50% of BMS patients complain of dry mouth (xerostomia) but do not exhibit measurable hyposalivation. The pain symptoms of BMS are invariably bilateral and are usually in multiple areas of the mouth. These symptoms often increase in intensity at the end of each day, and they seldom interfere with sleep. To be considered for BMS, the patient should have had the pain continuously for at least 4 to 6 months. Pain levels may vary from mild to severe, but moderate pain is the most frequent presentation. The pain should be described as daily bilateral oral burning (or pain-like) sensations deep within the oral mucosa, unremitting for at least 4 to 6 months. The symptoms should generally be continuous throughout the day and should not interfere with sleep.

Like many idiopathic diseases, BMS is a diagnosis made by a careful history and a thorough process of excluding other causes or diseases. Abnormalities that must be excluded include local pathology of the mucosal tissues, nutritional deficiencies (vitamin B_1, B_2, B_6, or B_{12}, folic acid), salivary hypofunction, and diabetic neuropathy. If any of these problems is discovered or if oral lesions are present, the diagnosis is not stomatopyrosis. The frequent observation of taste changes or sensory or chemosensory dysfunctions in BMS patients has suggested that this syndrome might reflect a neuropathic disorder [51]. The notion that BMS is due to psychogenic or psychosomatic factors has generally not been supported by scientific evidence [52,53]. However, many BMS patients exhibit high levels of anxiety and depression as well as pain relief after suitable administration of psychotropic drugs, such as antidepressants or benzodiazepines.

BMS treatment is still unsatisfactory, and there is no definitive cure. BMS patients have shown a good response to long-term therapy with systemic regimens of TCAs, gabapentin, or benzodiazepine-class drugs (anxiolytics). In a recent study, Gremeau-Richard et al [54] examined the effect of topical clonazepam in stomatodynia in a randomized placebo-controlled study. Their protocol required patients to suck a tablet of 1 mg of either clonazepam or placebo and hold their saliva near the pain sites in the mouth without swallowing for 3 minutes, then spit. This procedure was repeated three times a day for 14 days. The investigators included 48 patients (4 men and 44 women, aged 65 ± 2.1 years), and 41 completed the study. The reported decrease in pain intensity scores was 2.4 out of 10 (± 0.6) for clonazepam and only 0.6 out of 10 (± 0.4) for placebo. Not only was this a statistically significant difference but, more importantly, the blood concentration of clonazepam was relatively low with this method.

It is important to provide patients with information and reassurance about their condition. BMS subjects are likely to have consulted numerous specialists who stated that the mucosa was healthy, and may thus be convinced that their problems are imaginary. Patients must be made aware that their pain is "real," that the syndrome is common in middle-aged and elderly individuals, and that it is often linked to identified conditions. They must also be informed that the oral pain is not related to any form of cancer, that the treatment will be prolonged, and that not all the symptoms are sure to disappear. Avoidance of any triggering stimulants should be practiced (eg, smoking, spicy foods). Peri- and postmenopausal women with BMS should be referred to gynecologists to consider estrogen replacement therapy. Finally, BMS represents a disorder with a very poor prognosis in terms of quality of life, and the patient's lifestyle may worsen when psychologic dysfunctions occur [55].

Uncomfortable bite without obvious dental cause: occlusal dysesthesia

One final condition to be discussed here is occlusal dysesthesia [56]. The three most common complaints of patients with a persistently uncomfortable bite are "My bite is not comfortable," "My bite is off," and "I don't know where my teeth belong anymore." When such complaints surface, it is necessary to distinguish between those patients with true bite discrepancies and those with no observable abnormality of the occlusion. Most dentists with a few years of experience have experienced such a patient. Severe uncomfortable bite disorder patients are often given either a diagnosis of atypical facial pain or a psychiatric diagnosis, such as that of exaggerated somatic focus. One explanation for these complaints is that some individuals develop a sensitization of the mechanoreceptors in and around selected teeth, which produces an altered or even enhanced proprioceptive signaling from the teeth. This signaling produces an enhanced awareness of all mechanical stimulation. Unfortunately, this problem is fairly frequent and more likely to occur in the elderly. Gerstner et al [57] collected data using a survey (0–4 scale) that asked, "Do you have a problem with your bite being uncomfortable?" The data involved 127 consecutive TMJ clinic patients attending a university temporomandibular disorder (TMD) clinic for diagnosis and help with their jaw pain and dysfunction problems. Nearly 30% of the respondents scored 2 or higher on the question (Fig. 1). This study did not clarify the specific age of the patients who responded yes to the question, but, as mentioned, it is not uncommon to see this problem in an elderly population.

Sometimes, clear and demonstrable abnormality of the teeth, TMJ, or maxillomandibular relationship is present in these patients, and an immediate plan of correction can be made. In some cases, the complaint of bite discomfort develops spontaneously. When no occlusal abnormality or dentoalveolar pathology is evident, the confusion begins, and there are more opportunities for misadventure. For example, a dentist may attempt to make a good occlusion even better by performing occlusal adjustment of the teeth or by replacing the new dental restoration in the suspected tooth or teeth, hoping that the problem will simply resolve with time. If this measure fails, increasingly more aggressive and often irreversible interventions may follow. Unfortunately, these subsequent interventions may aggravate the patient's initial complaint. For example, Remick et al [58] described 21 patients with atypical facial pain who had undergone 65 dental or surgical treatments. Only one patient had less pain as a result of these treatments. The authors indicated in their case series that frequently a psychologic diagnosis was comorbid with the atypical facial pain and suggested that patients with this diagnosis should receive conservative dental and medical

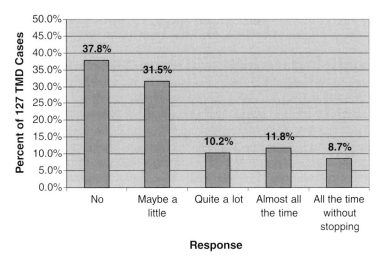

Fig. 1. Response to a question on bite comfort taken from a group of 127 consecutive clinic patients with TMD.

treatment and a behavioral assessment before dental and surgical procedures are contemplated. Although these cases were characterized as pain cases, the basic observation is equally applicable to patients with persistent uncomfortable bite without an observable occlusal abnormality.

Although many terms have been used in the past, including "phantom bite syndrome," Clark et al [59] suggested the term "occlusal dysesthesia" (OD) as the best one to describe the complaint of a persistently uncomfortable bite when a bite discrepancy cannot be observed. Occlusion is defined as the act of closure or the state of being closed. The dental meaning of the term "occlusion" relates to the static intercuspal relationship of the teeth and also to the act of closing the teeth. Dysesthesia can be described as a disagreeable or impaired (abnormal) sensation, whether spontaneous or evoked. OD is therefore defined as a "persistent uncomfortable sense of maximum intercuspation after all pulpal, periodontal, muscle and TMJ pathologies have been ruled out and a physically obvious bite discrepancy cannot be observed."

Two explanations for the phenomenon of OD (severe bite discomfort) are that patients have (1) a seriously altered oral kinesthetic ability or (2) a diagnosable psychiatric disorder. The kinesthetic ability of the jaw is defined as the tested accuracy of subjects to discriminate the position of the mandible in the path from maximum opening to maximum intercuspation. At least one theory attributes this disorder to a general loss of peripheral sensory receptor function in the jaw and teeth and, more specifically, to effects on the function of muscle spindles in the jaw closers. This theory is based on the report by Hellsing [60] that distortion of kinesthesia is independent of the amplitude and frequency of vibration to confound muscle spindle sensory afferents and persists during anesthesia of the TMJ and loading of the mandible. Hellsing also speculated that jaw muscle receptors may contribute to mandibular kinesthesia. Morimoto and Kawamura [61] also investigated mandibular kinesthesia and suggested that muscle spindles in jaw-closing muscles are primarily responsible for interdental thickness discrimination. Finally, van Duersen et al [62] showed that, with aging and associated peripheral neuropathy, the kinesthetic ability deteriorates. This group demonstrated that vibration had a greater effect on younger subjects, a reduced effect on the elderly, and an even smaller effect on those with peripheral neuropathy. This diminishing effect is presumably owing to the progressive dysfunction of the muscle spindles with aging and peripheral neuropathy, making them less relied on by the subjects.

Marbach [63] suggested that some subjects with phantom bite could instead have a neurotic disorder termed "dysmorphophobia." This is the belief that a body part is cosmetically defective in a person of normal appearance. In contrast, Greene and Gelb [64] reported on five subjects with what they termed proprioceptive dysfunction and symptoms enduring between 44 and 264 months. They found only one subject with a somatoform disorder; the other four "did not qualify for a psychopathological diagnosis, and certainly were not delusional or psychotic." Given this unresolved controversy, all occlusal dysesthesia cases warrant consideration for psychometric testing and psychologic evaluation. The primary psychologic disorder to be ruled out is somatoform disorder. The diagnostic condition somatoform disorder is also the most frequent diagnosis associated with a subjective sensory abnormality unconfirmed by objective signs and tests.

The treatment options for OD are (1) drug therapy, (2) psychotherapy, and (3) strategies to be used by the dentist to reduce mechanical stimulation of the sensitive area. Pimozide is one psychotomimetic drug that has been reported to be helpful in the treatment of phantom sensory phenomena. Pimozide is a nonphenothiazine neuroleptic drug similar in structure to haloperidol. It has many side effects that are problematic for the elderly, and even though positive somatic form behaviors have been noted within a week, it is still dangerous to use. Reports of up to 4.5 years of successful maintenance on pimozide are encouraging. More recently, resperidone has emerged as a preferred drug for complex problems like this one [65]. Patients with OD are reluctant to seek traditional psychotherapy, but the physician who has substantial suspicion of a somatoform disorder should obtain a psychiatric consultation and appropriate testing. No good direct treatment exists for idiopathic OD. The best symptomatic management, for those cases in which the complaint is localized to a single tooth or teeth in one region of the mouth, is to make the patient an occlusal disengagement device (eg, an anterior bite plane). Such a device allows the patient more or less to avoid contact on the offending posterior teeth. In such cases, when the disengagement splint is helpful, it is logical to reduce the thickness of the occlusal splint over several weeks or months until the posterior teeth come back into contact. No specific medication has been found helpful, other than a partially sedating medication (eg, clonazepam), which helps reduce anxiety and increase tolerance to the symptoms. The final and crucial component of treatment for OD is education. Specifically, it should be explained to patients that their complaints of a persistent uncomfortable bite often are not a physical problem but rather a mechanosensory disorder, which may best be characterized as the outward consequence of a pathologic alteration of the mandibular proprioceptive system. In these cases, mechanical therapies (eg, occlusal adjustment, restoration replacement) are not helpful, but it is hoped that, with time and symptomatic management, the severity of the problem will fade to a level of tolerance.

Summary

The actual prevalence of general pain in the elderly population is moderately high (ranging from 25% to 88%), and research suggests that 17.4% of the elderly will report one or more current or recent orofacial pains within a single year. Several causes of orofacial pain exist, including strong contraction-based movement disorders (such as dystonia and bruxism). Oral motor dysfunction is best managed with a multidisciplinary approach, including medications, protective devices (bite guards), and motor paralyzing injections (ie, botulinum toxin). One muscle condition that is more evident in the elderly than in younger patients is fibromyalgia. This chronic pain condition increases with age, affects up to 2% of the population, and is at least seven times more common in women. Several medications are used for FMS, but efficacy is low and tolerability remains a problem in the elderly. The best medications at present are the tricyclic medications (eg, nortriptyline), the sedative-hypnotics (zolpidem), and a weak opioid analgesic (tramadol). It is probably more important in the treatment of FMS that a physical medicine-behavioral treatment program be established and that the patient engage in daily physical exercise and relaxation.

Another cause of orofacial pain is temporal arteritis, which is commonly seen in older people; the mean age of onset is 70 years. Treatment of temporal arteritis usually involves corticosteroids in a dose sufficient to relieve symptoms. Approximately two thirds of headache pain in the elderly is caused by migraines or tension-type headaches, but when a new headache develops in the elderly, the other third may have an intracranial lesion or a systemic disease. The difficulty with headaches in the elderly is that the medications used in a younger cohort are problematic for many reasons. A frequently misdiagnosed disease in the elderly is TN. Once it is fully developed, it presents as a sudden, usually unilateral, severe, brief, stabbing, recurrent pain. In the early stages of the disease, it is often mistaken for a toothache due to dental abscess.

When the oral pain problem is a sustained pain in the teeth or gingival tissues, this condition is called atypical oral pain or atypical odontalgia;

once the tooth is extracted and the pain continues, the term "phantom tooth pain" is used. This disorder is most likely due to a long-lasting and perhaps permanent neuropathic alteration in the trigeminal nerve. Other oral neuropathic diseases that affect the elderly are postherpetic neuralgia, BMS, and an unusual disturbance in the patient's sense of bite comfort, described as OD. Suggested treatments for these neuropathic diseases have been described.

References

[1] Kane RL, Ouslander JG, Abrass IB. Essential of clinical geriatrics. 2nd edition. New York: McGraw-Hill; 1989.
[2] Ferrell BA, Ferrell BR, Osterweil D. Pain in the nursing home. J Am Geriatr Soc 1990;38(4): 409–14.
[3] Riley JL III, Gilbert GH, Heft MW. Orofacial pain symptom prevalence: selective sex differences in the elderly? Pain 1998;76(1–2):97–104.
[4] Bourgeois M, Bouilh P, Tignol J, et al. Spontaneous dyskinesias vs. neuroleptic-induced dyskinesias in 270 elderly subjects. J Nerv Ment Dis 1980;168(3):177–8.
[5] Fahn S, Marsden CD, Calne DB. Classification and investigation of dystonia. In: Marsden CD, Fahn S, editors. Movement disorders 2. London: Butterworths; 1987. p. 332–58.
[6] Vitale S, Miller NR, Mejico LJ, et al. A randomized, placebo-controlled, crossover clinical trial of super blue-green algae in patients with essential blepharospasm or Meige syndrome. Am J Ophthalmol 2004;138(1):18–32.
[7] Ransmayr G, Kleedorfer B, Dierckx RA, et al. Pharmacological study in Meige's syndrome with predominant blepharospasm. Clin Neuropharmacol 1988;11(1):68–76.
[8] Lavigne GJ, Montplaisir JY. Bruxism: epidemiology, diagnosis, pathophysiology and pharmacology. Adv Pain Res Ther 1995;21:387–404.
[9] Stubner S, Rustenbeck E, Grohmann R, et al. Severe and uncommon involuntary movement disorders due to psychotropic drugs. Pharmacopsychiatry 2004;37(Suppl 1):S54–64.
[10] Winocur E, Gavish A, Voikovitch M, et al. Drugs and bruxism: a critical review. J Orofac Pain 2003;17(2):99–111.
[11] Clark GT. The management of oromandibular motor disorders and facial spasms with intramuscular injections of botulinum toxin. Phys Med Rehabil Clin N Am 2003;14(4): 727–48.
[12] Gerwin RD. Classification, epidemiology, and natural history of myofascial pain syndrome. Curr Pain Headache Rep 2001;5(5):412–20.
[13] Shaver JL. Fibromyalgia syndrome in women. Nurs Clin North Am 2004;39(1):195–204.
[14] Staud R, Price DD, Robinson ME, et al. Maintenance of windup of second pain requires less frequent stimulation in fibromyalgia patients compared to normal controls. Pain 2004; 110(3):689–96.
[15] Cedraschi C, Desmeules J, Rapiti E, et al. Fibromyalgia: a randomised, controlled trial of a treatment programme based on self management. Ann Rheum Dis 2004;63(3):290–6.
[16] Altman R, Alarcon G, Appelrouth D, et al. The American College of Rheumatology criteria for the classification and reporting of osteoarthritis of the hand. Arthritis Rheum 1990; 33(11):1601–10.
[17] Rao SG, Bennett RM. Pharmacological therapies in fibromyalgia. Best Pract Res Clin Rheumatol 2003;17(4):611–27.
[18] Nielson WR, Jensen MP. Relationship between changes in coping and treatment outcome in patients with Fibromyalgia Syndrome. Pain 2004;109(3):233–41.
[19] Salvarani C, Cantini F, Boiardi L, et al. Polymyalgia rheumatica and giant-cell arteritis. N Engl J Med 2002;347(4):261–71.

[20] Frearson R, Cassidy T, Newton J. Polymyalgia rheumatica and temporal arteritis: evidence and guidelines for diagnosis and management in older people. Age Ageing 2003; 32(4):370–4.

[21] Gonzalez-Gay MA, Garcia-Porrua C, Amor-Dorado JC, et al. Influence of age, sex, and place of residence on clinical expression of giant cell arteritis in northwest Spain. J Rheumatol 2003;30(7):1548–51.

[22] Ellis ME, Ralston S. The ESR in the diagnosis and management of the polymyalgia rheumatica/giant cell arteritis syndrome. Ann Rheum Dis 1983;42(2):168–70.

[23] Hayreh SS, Zimmerman B. Visual deterioration in giant cell arteritis patients while on high doses of corticosteroid therapy. Ophthalmology 2003;110(6):1204–15.

[24] Solomon GD, Kunkel RS Jr, Frame J. Demographics of headache in elderly patients. Headache 1990;30(5):273–6.

[25] Waters WE. The Pontypridd headache survey. Headache 1974;14(2):81–90.

[26] Selby GW, Lance JW. Observations on 500 cases of migraine and allied vascular headache. J Neurol Neurosurg Psychiatry 1960;23:23–32.

[27] Wilkinson M. Clinical features of migraine. In: Vinken PJ, Bruyn GW, Klawans HL, et al, editors. Headache. New York: Elsevier; 1986. p. 117–83.

[28] Bronfort G, Nilsson N, Haas M, et al. Non-invasive physical treatments for chronic/recurrent headache. Cochrane Database Syst Rev 2004;3 CD001878.

[29] Zakrzewska JM. Diagnosis and differential diagnosis of trigeminal neuralgia. Clin J Pain 2002;18(1):14–21.

[30] Headache Classification Committee of the International Headache Society. Classification and diagnostic criteria for headache disorders, cranial neuralgias and facial pain. Cephalalgia 1988;8(Suppl 7):1–96.

[31] Sindrup SH, Jensen TS. Pharmacotherapy of trigeminal neuralgia. Clin J Pain 2002;18(1): 22–7.

[32] Harris M. Psychogenic aspects of facial pain. Br Dent J 1974;136:199–202.

[33] Rees RT, Harris M. Atypical odontalgia. Br J Oral Surg 1979;16:212–8.

[34] Graff-Radford SB, Solberg WK. Atypical odontalgia. J Craniomandib Disord 1992;6: 260–5.

[35] Reik L Jr. Atypical odontalgia: a localized form of atypical facial pain. Headache 1984;24: 222–4.

[36] Kreisberg MK. Atypical odontalgia: differential diagnosis and treatment. J Am Dent Assoc 1982;104:852–4.

[37] Brooke RI. Atypical odontalgia. A report of twenty-two cases. Oral Surg Oral Med Oral Pathol 1980;49:196–9.

[38] Marbach JJ. Phantom tooth pain. J Endod 1978;4:362–72.

[39] Billet J, Kerebel B, Lumineau JP, et al. A rare dental abnormality: the phantom tooth. Apropos of a case. Rev Stomatol Chir Maxillofac 1975;76:23–31.

[40] Reisner H. Atypical neuralgias of the head and face. Zahnarztl Mitt (German) 1976;66: 1153–6.

[41] Reisner H. Phantom pain in dentistry (phantom tooth). Osterr Z Stomatol 1977;74: 423–7.

[42] Merskey H, Bogduk N. Classification of chronic pain: descriptions of chronic pain syndromes and definitions of pain terms. 2nd edition. Seattle (WA): IASP Press; 1994.

[43] Marbach JJ. Is phantom tooth pain a deafferentation (neuropathic) syndrome? Part I: Evidence derived from pathophysiology and treatment. Oral Surg Oral Med Oral Pathol 1993;75(1):95–105.

[44] Johnson RW, Dworkin RH. Treatment of herpes zoster and postherpetic neuralgia. BMJ 2003;326(7392):748–50.

[45] Schmader K. Herpes zoster in older adults. Clin Infect Dis 2001;32(10):1481–6.

[46] Dworkin RH, Nagasako EM, Johnson RW, et al. Acute pain in herpes zoster: the famciclovir database project. Pain 2001;94(1):113–9.

[47] Stranska R, Schuurman R, de Vos M, et al. Routine use of a highly automated and internally controlled real-time PCR assay for the diagnosis of herpes simplex and varicella-zoster virus infections. J Clin Virol 2004;30(1):39–44.

[48] Van Doornum GJ, Guldemeester J, Osterhaus AD, et al. Diagnosing herpes virus infections by real-time amplification and rapid culture. J Clin Microbiol 2003;41(2):576–80.

[49] Nicholson BD. Diagnosis and management of neuropathic pain: a balanced approach to treatment. J Am Acad Nurse Pract 2003;15(Suppl 12):3–9.

[50] Marbach JJ. Medically unexplained chronic orofacial pain. Temporomandibular pain and dysfunction syndrome, orofacial phantom pain, burning mouth syndrome, and trigeminal neuralgia. Med Clin North Am 1999;83(3):691–710.

[51] List T, Axelsson S, Leijon G. Pharmacologic interventions in the treatment of temporomandibular disorders, atypical facial pain, and burning mouth syndrome. A qualitative systematic review. J Orofac Pain 2003;17(4):301–10.

[52] Zakrzewska JM, Forssell H, Glenny AM. Interventions for the treatment of burning mouth syndrome: a systematic review. J Orofac Pain 2003;17(4):293–300.

[53] Scala A, Checchi L, Montevecchi M, et al. Update on burning mouth syndrome: overview and patient management. Crit Rev Oral Biol Med 2003;14(4):275–91.

[54] Gremeau-Richard C, Woda A, Navez ML, et al. Topical clonazepam in stomatodynia: a randomised placebo-controlled study. Pain 2004;108(1–2):51–7.

[55] Buchanan J, Zakrzewska J. Burning mouth syndrome. Clin Evid 2002;7:1239–43.

[56] Clark GT, Simmons M. Occlusal dysesthesia and temporomandibular disorders: is there a link? Alpha Omegan 2003;96(2):33–9.

[57] Gerstner GE, Clark GT, Goulet JP. Validity of a brief questionnaire in detecting temporomandibular disorders. Community Dent Oral Epidemiol 1994;22:235–42.

[58] Remick RA, Blasberg B, Barton JS, et al. Ineffective dental and surgical treatment associated with atypical facial pain. Oral Surg Oral Med Oral Pathol 1983;55:355–8.

[59] Clark GT, Tsukiyama Y, Baba K, et al. The validity and utility of disease detection methods and of occlusal therapy for temporomandibular disorders. Oral Surg Oral Med Oral Pathol Oral Radiol Endod 1997;83:101–6.

[60] Hellsing G. Distortion of mandibular kinesthesia induced by vibration of human jaw muscles. Scand J Dent Res 1978;86:486–94.

[61] Morimoto T, Kawamura Y. Conditioning-effect of vibratory stimulation on dimension discrimination of objects held between human tooth arches. Arch Oral Biol 1976;21:219–20.

[62] van Deursen RW, Sanchez MM, Ulbrecht JS, et al. The role of muscle spindles in ankle movement perception in human subjects with diabetic neuropathy. Exp Brain Res 1998; 120:1–8.

[63] Marbach JJ. Psychological factors for failure to adapt to dental prostheses. Dent Clin North Am 1985;29:215–33.

[64] Greene PA, Gelb M. Proprioception dysfunction vs. phantom bite: diagnostic considerations reported. TM Diary 1994;2:16–7.

[65] Elmer KB, George RM, Peterson K. Therapeutic update: use of risperidone for the treatment of monosymptomatic hypochondriacal psychosis. J Am Acad Dermatol 2000; 43(4):683–6.

ELSEVIER
SAUNDERS

THE DENTAL
CLINICS
OF NORTH AMERICA

Dent Clin N Am 49 (2005) 363–376

Underserved Elderly Issues in the United States: Burdens of Oral and Medical Health Care

Veronica A. Greene, DDS, MPH

University of Southern California, School of Dentistry, 925 West 34th Street, Los Angeles, CA 90089-0641, USA

Several recent national reports, such as the Institute of Medicine report on Understanding and Eliminating Racial and Ethnic Disparities in Health Care (March 2002) [1,2], the US Surgeon General Report on Oral Health in America (May 2000) [3], and the National Call to Action Initiative (May 2003) [4], have highlighted the disparate quality and extent of health care services received by racial and ethnic minorities in the United States. The gaps in health care services vary by race or ethnicity, income stratum, age, and area of residence (urban versus nonurban) [5–10]. Low income, lack of supplemental insurance, and age of 85 years or greater are other risk factors for poor access and use of health care [5,7,8]. Some prospective studies conducted in the United States and other nations demonstrate racial disparities in receipt of services that are not explained by differences in access or disease severity [11–13]. Even when one controlled for socio-economic differences, many of these disparities remained [8,13]. Hence, these disparities in health care may be attributable to multiple longstanding factors, one or more of which may be confounded by other factors [13]. Although most of these reports charge their readers with reducing or eliminating these disparities, effective strategies must target every level of the health care system, including cross-cultural training, regulatory and policy interventions (eg, national consensus on best practices, using evidence-based guidelines), and financing [14].

This article focuses primarily on African Americans, Hispanics, and American Indians or Alaskan Natives. Although several other racial or ethnic groups have experienced disparate health care access or disease burden in the United States, most research and data collected by Summary

E-mail address: vgreene@usc.edu

Health Statistics (surveys administered by the US Department of Health and Human Services) were not available for these groups, particularly distinct subgroups of Asian Americans. Distinctive cultural influences, traditions, and belief systems, as well as genetic or hereditary factors of disease, are observed among certain subgroups. Current and future oral health research should strive to assess these trends among and within distinct subgroups of racial or ethnic populations to identify successful strategies to eliminate or reduce these health care disparities.

Rationale for targeting older Americans

As of the year 2000, the elderly represented about 12.4% of the general population [15], yet their health care expenditure gross national product (GNP) was approximately 14% in 2003 [16]. In 1996, the annual range was from $8,742 per capita as a group to $38,906 per capita for the institutionalized elderly [7]. By 2000, total health care expenses for those 65 years of age or older approached $204 million, compared with about $424 million for those less than 65 years of age [17]. Although most of the elderly have some form of medical insurance (89%) [11,18], only about 22% have dental insurance [7,19]. Census projections for the year 2030 predict that there will be 54 to 56 million Americans aged 65 years or older, with an expected health care GNP of 25% [7,15].

Older Americans' health status has shown improvements over the past decade [6], yet there are tremendous gaps in the health care services received by this population [1,2,5]. Although most older Americans have either Medicare or private health insurance, many live alone, and barriers such as chronic illness, social distraction, poor literacy, cultural practices, and even mental disorders limit their access to Medicare and their ability to navigate the health care maze [8–11,14].

In 2000, 0.9% of the United States population self-identified as American Indians or Alaskan Natives (AI/ANs), with another 1.5% identifying themselves as combined AI/AN and one other race or ethnicity [15]. It is generally accepted that American Indians and Alaskan Natives have a higher burden of disease, injury, and premature mortality than non-Hispanic whites [20]. Average life expectancy among AI/ANs has increased 39% over the past 5 decades [21]. The Indian Health Service (IHS) has been credited with surveillance and interventions for infectious and chronic diseases among AI/ANs [21]. These interventions are reported to have contributed to the improved health outcomes in this population since the 1980s [22]. However, Katz [20] reports that IHS may not be an adequate source of care for most AI/ANs and that pervasive disparities within this subgroup may go unrecognized. Others have reported troubling gaps in health care access and use, insurance coverage, and income among various subgroups of AI/ANs, even among those receiving care from the IHS.

Trends in quality of care also show significant disparities among older minority Americans and those with functional limitations or disabilities requiring long-term or home health care, palliative care, pain management, hospice care, or even preventive care (eg, adult immunizations) [6,23]. Over the past decade, the number of elderly persons with disabilities has declined; their access to disability benefits has been better than that of nonelderly low-income persons [6]. Disabled older minority persons report more problems with quality of care (11%) than do whites (4%), yet blacks and Hispanics (12%) are less likely than whites (20%) to report delays in access to care due to costs [6,8,16]. Within nursing homes, there are racial disparities among older adults receiving influenza or pneumococcal immunizations, pain management, and rehabilitative care, even with equitable insurance coverage [6,8,9,11].

The gap among older Americans is even wider for dental care, where demand for services trails need. In addition to lacking resources for this perceived optional health care [19,24], most elderly people are more concerned about basic necessities, such as maintaining shelter, food, and prescription medications [8]. Hence, the dental profession should improve its role and responsibility in caring for the elderly by (1) improving understanding of the relationship between oral and systemic health [6,25], (2) broadening cultural competence to close the gaps between available, accessible, and acceptable oral and dental care [3,4,26], and (3) marketing or promoting high-quality continuous dental care for this expanding and needy subpopulation [6,8,27].

History of disparities in health care

The Civil Rights Act (1964) prohibits discrimination by institutions receiving federal funds, and the Medicare and Medicaid Act (1965) reduced financial barriers to care for minority and nonminority elderly low-income Americans [8,9]. Nonetheless, health care among older underrepresented racial and ethnic populations still differs from that of the majority population, and these disparities have not been explained by factors such as access, insurance status, needs or preferences, or type of interventions or services [5,9].

In fact, several studies and clinical trials reported fewer underrepresented minorities receiving preventive care (eg, cancer screening), cardiac care or surgery, diabetes management, and home health or rehabilitative nursing care [10,12,13,18]. However, more of these individuals received aggressive irreversible surgeries (eg, amputation, bilateral orchiectomy) or experienced poor outcomes from coronary events, cardiac surgery, or cancer or diabetes treatment [5,8,12,13].

These different subgroups have variable needs among, within, and across communities, ethnicities, and income strata [1,2,6,8]. Thus, viable solutions must also identify specific and multiple factors that contribute to these disparities.

These health care disparities have been recognized for decades [6], but only within the past 20 years has there been demonstrable national response. The Clinton administration's 1998 Initiative on Race was the broadest, resulting in the Health and Human Services Racial and Ethnic Health Disparities Initiative [1,2,6,28]. During the last decade, federal agencies have actively supported research aimed at reducing health disparities in minority populations, including biomedical, behavioral, and evidence-based clinical research activities [28]. These activities have yielded the national reports cited in this article: Healthy People 2010, Oral Health in America, the National Call to Action Initiative, the Institute of Medicine reports, and a recently developed Regional Research Center on Minority Oral Health in Los Angeles, California, supported by the National Institute of Dental and Craniofacial Research [28].

Older Americans and oral health status

Over the past few decades, growth among Americans over the age of 65 years has surpassed expectations [3,15]. By 2030, this age cohort will account for almost one third of the United States population and will significantly burden the health care system [7]. As with medical care, the oral and dental needs of the elderly vary widely and according to similar factors [6,19]. Although the majority are likely to retain teeth throughout their lifespan, routine dental care and screening for oral disease will increase either demand for access or use of dental care services by elderly subgroups [4,29].

Subsidized medical versus dental care

Medicaid, a jointly funded federal–state program for eligible low-income persons and the disabled low-income elderly, provides limited reimbursements for selected dental care in some states [11,30]. Poor elderly, therefore, may not even seek dental care because of socioeconomic constraints [24,29]. These poor elderly tend to be overrepresented by racial and ethnic minorities [8,9,30]. Limited resources and inability to pay may be among several factors that explain poor access to preventive or routine dental care among these underserved elderly. Patients' perception of need and, often, patients' and providers' poor understanding of the associations between oral health and systemic disease also contribute to inadequate health promotion and referral [3,4,30].

Dental use services

Use of dental services by the elderly correlates with dental insurance or income status; only 22% had private dental insurance in 1995, and most of these services were paid for "out of pocket" [19,31]. One dental visit per year, a measure of use, was reported by 54% of all elders surveyed in 1997 [7,19]. However, when the elders were asked how often they visited the dentist, that proportion varied from 37% of those with teeth to 75% of those without teeth [19].

A modified survey, administered in 2002, yielded more useful data on access. Of a representative sample of elderly persons aged 65 years or older, 48.4% of those who had private insurance had visited the dentist or dental health provider within the previous 6 months, as had 48% of those with Medicaid, Medicare, or no insurance [16]. An additional 38% reported no dental visit for more than 5 years, and 2% reported never having visited a dentist [16].

Untreated dental caries

Several recent reports indicate that almost one third of the elderly have untreated caries or periodontal disease [3,19]. The prevalence of dental disease (caries, missing teeth, periodontal disease, and oropharyngeal cancer) is disproportionately greater among the African American and Hispanic elderly [30]. In 2001, Vargas et al [19] reported that 47% of African American elders had untreated dental disease; adding poverty to the equation increased the proportion to 50%.

Comparisons from sampling over 3-year intervals spanning 3 decades (National Health and Nutritional Examination Survey [NHANES] I–III) [16] showed little overall change in the proportion of 65 to 74 year olds with untreated dental caries: 29.7% (1971–1974) versus 25.4% (1988–1994). However, blacks had worse caries, changing from 41.5% to 46.7% over the same survey period. Hispanics were surveyed only in the last 2 decades, 1982 to 1984 and 1988 to 1994, but they showed negligible improvement, from 44.3% to 43.8% [16]. Among these minority elders, being "near poor" as opposed to "poor" (ie, below the federal poverty threshold) was associated with fewer untreated dental caries: 22.7% for whites and 43.6% for blacks, whereas 39% of the white poor and 50% of the black poor had untreated caries [16].

The percentage of edentulism in 2002 was 24% for all persons between 65 and 74 years old and 32.5% for those aged 75 years or greater [7]. These proportions varied by insurance status for those over the age of 65 years: 24% of those with private insurance were edentulous, compared with 45.4% of those with Medicaid or Medicare, 31.8% of those with Medicare only, 34% of those with another insurance source, and 29.2% of the uninsured [16]. In the NHANES III survey of noninstitutionalized elderly between the ages of 65 to 74 years, 46.7% of blacks and 43.8% of Mexican Americans were edentulous, compared with 22.7% of whites [7]. More data about health status and less about oral health were available for AI/ANs. However, the 2002 National Health Interview Survey reported that 29.2% of AI/ANs at least 18 years old had visited a dentist in the past 6 months,

13.9% had not seen a dentist in more than 5 years, and 1.2% reported never having visited a dentist [16]. In this minority group, the rate of edentulism (8.6%) was reported for all adults in 2002, without age stratification [16].

Periodontal disease

Along with dental caries, periodontal disease is more prevalent among adults and children the lower socioeconomic strata of United States adults and children. Nutritional status may be adversely affected by these socio-economic factors [28]. Because racial and ethnic minorities are dispropor-tionately affected by each of these factors, we see a higher prevalence of gingivitis (Mexican Americans), general periodontitis (blacks), caries, and edentulism among these subpopulations [16]. At least 36% of lower-socioeconomic-status adults over 75 years of age have moderate to severe periodontal disease [28]. According to the Centers for Disease Control and Prevention, 23% of all 65 to 74 year olds have severe periodontitis [30].

A Finnish group reported increasing retention of teeth in the expanding subgroup of elderly in all industrialized nations [32]. In a population-based Helsinki Ageing Study, a cohort of 65 to 75 year olds were assessed and treated between 1990 and 1991 [32]. Because most of these elders retained about 50% of their natural dentition, establishing and maintaining a healthy periodontium was the goal of the investigators. A small percentage of these elders had no signs of periodontal disease, but the vast majority required scaling and root planning, and at least 11% needed complex periodontal procedures. Overall, as a group, their need for frequent or complex therapy was very low [32]. American and British investigators have reported similar findings about periodontal health in the elderly who retained their teeth [33–35].

IHS's primary care providers have reported two major comorbid conditions that appear to magnify dental and periodontal disease among older AI/ANs: type II diabetes and long-term tobacco use [36]. These adults had 2% edentulism (complete) and 60% untreated caries; the rates varied widely by state or region. Risk factors included smoking and smokeless tobacco use, high consumption of refined sugar, diabetes, and infrequent dental care. Elders were defined as those of at least 55 years of age, of whom 23% had no remaining upper teeth and 20% had no dentures. Root caries was common in 33%, even though the overall percentage with untreated caries was about 60%. These providers found that periodontal disease was underestimated because of high tooth loss. The lowest percentage of advanced periodontitis was in Alaska, and this figure was still three times the national average (for adults at least 35 years old) [36]. Results of NHANES III reflected 8.6% edentulism among AI/ANs aged at least 18 years as of 2002; these data were not stratified by age greater than or equal to 65 years [16].

Oral cancer

With the exception of oral cancer, dental disease is not usually life-threatening. Hence, many policymakers do not appreciate the need for dental care as a priority when appropriating limited health care resources [3,19]. Racial and ethnic minorities are disproportionately affected by oropharyngeal cancer, from staging of diagnosis through 5-year survival [7,28,37].

Even though younger African American men have the highest incidence and worst prognosis, older men in this racial and ethnic group are similarly overrepresented [7,28,37]. In 1990, oral/pharyngeal cancer incidence for United States males was 18.7% (white), 26.1% (black), 15.1% (Asian), and 10.9% (Hispanic). By 1999, the incidence declined by 2.2% to 2.7% in every group except black and Hispanic males, whose incidence varied each year (blacks) or increased by 0.9% (Hispanics) [7]. Overall, as of 2002, 56% of elderly whites and 34% of blacks survived oral cancer at 5 years following diagnosis [30]. Five-year survival relative rates were available for blacks and whites only over a 25-year period. White males showed a 3.4% improved survival rate between 1974 and 1998 (54.4% versus 57.8%), whereas the rate for black males showed a slight decline, from 31.2% to 29.5%, over the same period [7,28].

Racial differences in survival often are explained by stage at diagnosis, as in the work of Brazilian investigators Franco et al and several previously published American studies [37]. However, despite diagnosis at a similar stage, blacks still had poorer survival than whites with oral or pharyngeal cancers [37]. In the North Carolina cohort, study subjects ranged from 14 to 108 years old; however, 17.8% were aged at least 75 years, and 56% were aged between 55 and 74 years. Survival was assessed over 18 months following diagnosis of oral or pharyngeal cancer; blacks died at a relative rate of 7.1% compared with whites (4.5%) within the first 2 months [37]. From 3 to 18 months, blacks still had about twice the hazard of whites for localized tumors; pharyngeal sites had eight times greater hazard than did oral sites [37].

A recent report of cancer rates among AI/AN reflects a lower mortality, 161.4 per 100,000 population, than the United States rate for all racial and ethnic minorities combined (205.5 per 100,000) [21]. Although oral/pharyngeal cancer was not among the top 10 types of cancer in this minority group, an average life expectancy of 71 years (1995) [21] and improved oral health care services (eg, early screening) should result in a low incidence of oral/pharyngeal cancer if key risk factors are significantly reduced—such as chronic use of alcohol and tobacco, especially in selected tribal regions [21,22].

Socioeconomic disparities

Socioeconomic status (SES) is a useful measure but is often complicated to ascertain. NHANES III used a composite index (measure) derived from individual education achievement and family income relative to poverty threshold [38]. SES is reported to be associated with differential health outcomes across societies [33,39] or on a gradient (lower SES associated with worse health outcomes; higher SES with better outcomes) [38]. Drury et al [38] assessed adults (>18 years) for indicators of oral disease or need for dental restorations. Lower SES (24%) was associated with a higher proportion of untreated dental caries (49.9%), more edentulism and gingivitis, and limited root canal therapy (2.4%). The investigators found that racial and ethnic minority status intensified these effects; SES interacted with race and ethnicity, particularly for edentulism. Although the elderly were not well represented in their sample, the investigators' findings implied similar or more pronounced disparities among older Americans [38].

The International Collaborative Study of Oral Outcomes-II USA Ethnicity and Aging Research Project evaluated population sociodemographic characteristics and dental care delivery in several communities: Native Americans in urban or rural locations, with and without fluoridated water, and Hispanic and African American communities across the United States [22,40]. Challenges in delivery of dental care were found to be diverse and often unique, varying by location, source of finances, type of provider or provider setting, and available special services [22]. SES indicators selected by this group included proportion of adults with a high school diploma, per capita income, and proportion of residents employed [22]. In only one of the study locations, near a dental school in Baltimore, was there a dental treatment project specifically for the elderly; African American elderly were overrepresented and were more likely to have unmet needs [22].

A Florida Dental Care Study assessed the oral health status of 724 persons of different ages, genders, and races or ethnicities [39]. The group conducted phone interviews to document self-reports of pain over various orofacial sites, along with other subjective ratings [39]. Comparing their findings with other studies that evaluated the association of SES with perceptions of health, predictors of behavior, and other lifestyle-related factors, the authors described the limitations of some of these studies [39]. For example, one study used composite measures of subjective oral health to demonstrate an association with SES among disadvantaged Hispanic and African American adults [24], whereas another reported SES as a predictor of avoidance of certain oral habits [39].

Among elderly patients in the Florida Dental Care Study, black or African American race or ethnicity was the only significant predictor of orofacial pain (tooth- and non–tooth-related) in multivariate analyses that included factors such as poverty status, lack of dental insurance, and lower educational attainment [39]. The authors cited studies conducted in Sweden, Canada, and the United States that found no associations between toothache or jaw pain and SES, and others that reported strong associations [39].

Demand for oral and dental care is neither equitably distributed across SES nor explained by cost of care among the elderly [41]. A cohort study using data from insurance claims assessed multiple variables (eg, pharmacy use, medical visits, lab services) relevant to health care in a comparison of dental users with nonusers. Most elders in this group consistently had low use of oral health care services over their lifespans. Minority elders, particularly African Americans with moderate education, were twice as likely as whites to participate in a program offering a waiver of fees for dental care. This finding suggests that eliminating financial barriers to oral health care would affect use of these services, even among minorities with moderately high income or educational status [41].

Impact on quality of life and longevity

With the goal of improving quality of life and sustaining healthier lives as life expectancy increases, we must engage all resources to prepare for future productivity. By 2011, today's middle-aged baby boomers will be elderly (>65 years), and their demands for high quality of life will require expansion of social and health care services [42]. Disease prevention, health promotion, and independent lifestyles are major requirements for high quality of life. Health care expenditure for tomorrow's elderly is expected to reach 25% by 2030 [42]. Aging is usually associated with chronic or disabling disorders and increased morbidity [8]. Preventing or reducing morbidity may be one of the best proactive methods of keeping health care costs down, not only for ambulatory and inpatient hospital care but also for long-term care [42]. Health promotion programs that seek out the elderly to teach them self-management and injury prevention or to provide them with early screening will likely yield better outcomes and reduced morbidity [8]. Although Medicare covers preventive services, only about 10% of the elderly receive recommended screening and immunizations [7,42].

Measuring the impact of oral health on quality of life may be a cost-effective and invaluable strategy. A national survey in the United Kingdom assessed oral health disparities among a random probability sample of households in 1999 [43]. Several factors (n = 16) related to oral health status were categorized as physical, social, or psychologic, and their impact on quality of life was stratified by good, bad, or no effect among the adults surveyed, only 23% of whom were aged at least 65 years [42]. Although 73% of all respondents perceived that oral health did affect their quality of life, physical attributes weighed more heavily with them than social or psychologic ones (eg, smiling, laughing, confidence). Higher social status or income was a significant predictor of the impact of oral health status on quality of life, but the most predictable positive oral health indicator was the retention of teeth without the need for dentures [42].

Discussion

Health care outcomes are influenced by an individual's timely access to essential services, ability to pay for services, understanding of signs or symptoms, and need to seek care. Other factors (eg, belief system, trust in providers or offered interventions) and comorbid conditions have been identified as potential barriers [8,9,44]. Evidence-based research has demonstrated strong links between the development of oral/pharyngeal cancers and the chronic use (and dose-response relationship) of tobacco and alcohol [16,30,37,42]. Early detection and treatment are associated with greater proportional survival [16,30,37]. Hence, screening campaigns not only need to be broadened but to be targeted to racial or ethnic groups with specific high-risk behaviors, whose members still may be unaware of these associations.

During the twenty-first century, health care services will be in greater demand as the graying of Americans proceeds and as better-educated consumers seek specific care [31]. Oral health services have not been well used by those with greatest need or worst health status [25,31]. Use of dental care is attributable to factors other than manpower and access; beliefs about oral health, personal practices, national agenda, financial resources, and health professionals' commitment to improving the system are at least equally important [22,40]. Dental health care professionals should become better equipped to treat underserved populations and to adopt partnerships that expand financial resources to cover essential costs of oral and dental care for the needy, especially the elderly [25,31].

Several strategic plans have been echoed by many research investigators, educators, and communities [8,9,45]. Multiple disciplines of health professional educators and institutions consistently working together to reduce disparities should positively affect these shortages at the primary and secondary levels: namely, the education and training of health professionals and the delivery of basic health care [2,31,45].

Although medical care is not optimally distributed, the dentist-to-population ratio in several areas of the United States is even worse [31]; it is grossly inadequate to meet the needs of many underserved communities [46]. Government has traditionally taken the primary responsibility for reducing shortages, eliminating disparities, and providing resources to train more providers for hardship areas. However, successful expansion of quality health care for needy subpopulations requires multilevel commitment by stakeholders (providers, policymakers, communities, and consumers) [46]. All stakeholders must share the tasks of targeted health promotion, advocacy, and lobbying for better distribution of resources to improve coverage, access, and availability of culturally representative providers.

Instead of practicing traditional roles in segregated disciplines, health professionals could serve multiple roles. For instance, a specialist diagnostician who screens for signs of disorders affecting selected organs could then play the "gatekeeper" in directing families immediately to other disciplines for assessment and care of the detected disorder [45]. Sharing expertise between medical and dental health care professionals serving high-risk families and communities has shown promising success (eg, a pediatric oral screening and prevention campaign: dental caries assessment and referral concurrent with Immunization Outreach) [45].

Prevention and management of dental disease among the elderly may continue to be a challenge over the next decade, particularly in underserved communities. The many tiers of intervention required to eliminate these disparities are distinct in certain areas but interactive in others. The fundamental approach—primary prevention and education—could be simple to implement jointly with medical screening programs for the elderly. Community-level outreach involving culturally representative staff or culturally sensitized professionals is essential to overcoming barriers such as belief systems (eg, oral health is insignificant) and problems in personal motivation (eg, concerns about expense, lower priority given to oral health, misunderstanding of the impact of oral health on overall health, nutrition, and aesthetics).

Despite ongoing initiatives, progress is slow toward eliminating racial and ethnic disparities in the United States, particularly in oral health. Racial and ethnic disparities persist among the 10 leading indicators identified in Healthy People 2010 Objectives [16,28,45]. Whether one looks at chronic disorders common to aging populations or at the provision of essential preventive or intervention services, the experiences and outcomes of racial and ethnic minority elders are still distinct [21,44].

Communication can be improved through provider behavior changes, including the motivation to become culturally competent, and through media-driven community-level health education [1,5]. Economic factors that influence health insurance coverage or ability to pay for noncovered services must be favorable to the implementation of policy changes. Expanding the eligibility for broad coverage, particularly when it is deemed a "medical necessity," may greatly affect access to care. If managed care, as we now know it, were established as "prospective" reimbursement for medically necessary dental care, the most vulnerable populations would be able to receive essential services [2,25,31]. Otherwise, financial incentives (eg, broader provider's professional tax relief) might offset many nonreimbursed fees to promote routine screening for subpopulations with greater risk factors for oral disease.

Older Americans and racial and ethnic minorities, as separate risk populations, may experience some similar challenges that perpetuate health care disparities. Reducing or eliminating these inequities will probably require an attack on known barriers to access, consistent efforts to dispel misperceptions of health and disease, mistrust, and other detrimental belief systems, and an easing of financial constraints. Perhaps we need to declare a national moratorium to ensure equitable access and quality primary care for all. Another option may be to implement a functional, universally accepted health system that addresses special needs of the currently high-risk subpopulations without compromising coverage limits for the terminally ill. In essence, the best goal may be to prioritize coverage for the most needy at the primary level, with the long-term goal of reducing costs at the tertiary level.

Proposal: a 5-year implementation and corresponding evaluation plan for such a health system could be developed. Not only would this plan serve to correct what we have experienced as failures in health care delivery, while prospectively budgeting for comprehensive health care for the underserved elderly, but it could measure efficacy and cost-effectiveness of primary prevention and early intervention for the medical and dental needs of one of the nation's most vulnerable subpopulations. Then, the Healthy People 2020 Objectives may be strikingly less monumental to achieve.

References

[1] Hurtado MP, Swift EK, Corrigon JM, editors. Institute of Medicine. Committee on the National Quality Report on Health Care Delivery. Envisioning the National Healthcare Quality Report. Washington, DC: National Academies Press; 2001.

[2] Smedley BD, Stith AY, Nelson AR, editors. Unequal treatment: confronting racial and ethnic disparities in health care. Washington (DC): The National Academies Press; 2003.

[3] US Department of Health and Human Services. Public Health Service. Oral health in America: a report of the Surgeon General. Rockville (MD): US Department of Health and Human Services, National Institute of Dental and Craniofacial Research, National Institutes of Health; 2000.

[4] US Department of Health and Human Services. A national call to action to promote oral health. Rockville (MD): US Department of Health and Human Services, Public Health Service, Centers for Disease Control and Prevention, National Institutes of Health, National Institute of Dental and Craniofacial Research; 2003. Publication #NIH 03–5303.

[5] Nelson AR. Unequal treatment: report of the Institute of Medicine on racial and ethnic disparities in healthcare. Ann Thorac Surg 2003;76:S1377–81.

[6] US Department of Health and Human Services, Agency for Healthcare Research and Quality. National Healthcare Disparities Report. Rockville (MD): US Department of Health and Human Services; 2003.

[7] Fried VM, Prager K, MacKay AP, et al. Chartbook on trends in the health of Americans. Health, United States, 2003. Hyattsville (MD): National Center for Health Statistics; 2003.

[8] Larkin VM, Alston RJ, Middleton RA, et al. Underrepresented ethnically and racially diverse aging populations with disabilities: trends and recommendations. J Rehabil 2003; 69(2):26–32.

[9] Lillie-Blanton M, Brodie M, Rowland D, et al. Race, ethnicity, and the health care system: public perceptions and experiences. Med Care Res Rev 2000;57(Suppl 1):218–35.

[10] Weinick RM, Zuvekas SH, Cohen JW. Racial and ethnic differences in access to and use of health care services, 1977 to 1996. Med Care Res Rev 2000;57(Suppl 1):36–54.

[11] Zukevas SH, Taliaferro GS. Pathways to access: health insurance, the health care delivery system, and racial/ethnic disparities, 1996–1999. Health Aff 2003;22(3):139–53.

[12] LaVeist TA, Nickerson KJ, Bowie JV. Attitudes about racism, medical mistrust, and satisfaction with care among African American and white cardiac patients. Med Care Res Rev 2000;57(Suppl 1):146–61.

[13] Laditka JN. Hazards of hospitalization for ambulatory care sensitive conditions among older women: evidence of greater risks for African Americans and Hispanics. Med Care Res Rev 2003;60(4):468–95.

[14] Mold JW, Fryer GE, Thomas CH. Who are the uninsured elderly in the United States? J Am Geriatr Soc 2004;52:601–6.

[15] US Census Bureau. Census 2000 summary file 1: 1990 census of population, general population characteristics, United States (1990 CP-1-1). Available at: http://factfinder.census.gov/servlet/. Accessed July 2004.

[16] Centers for Disease Control and Prevention. NationalCenter for Health Statistics. Summary health statistics for US adults: National Health Interview Survey 2002. I. Vital Health Stat 10 2004;222:14,148–9. DHHS Public #(PHS) 2004–1550.

[17] Langa KM, Fendrick AM, Chernew ME, et al. Out-of-pocket health-care expenditures among older Americans with cancer. Value Health 2004;7(2):186–94.

[18] Monheit AC. Race/ethnicity and health insurance status: 1987–1996. Med Care Res Rev 2000;57(Suppl 1):11–25.

[19] Vargas CM, Kramarow EA, Yellowitz JA. The oral health of older Americans. Aging Trends 2001;3:1–8.

[20] Katz RJ. Addressing the health care needs of American Indians and Alaska Natives. J Am Public Health 2004;94(1):13–5.

[21] Centers for Disease Control and Prevention. Health disparities experienced by American Indians and Alaska Natives. MMWR Morbid Mortal Wkly Rep 2003;52(30): 699–702.

[22] Reifel NM, Davidson PL, Rana H, et al. ICS-II USA research locations: environmental, dental care delivery system, and population sociodemographic characteristics. Adv Dent Res 1997;11(2):210–6.

[23] Rosenbaum S, Markus A. US civil rights policy and access to health care by minority Americans: implications for a changing health care system. Med Care Res Rev 2000; 57(Suppl 1):236–59.

[24] Atchison KA, Gift HC. Perceived oral health in a diverse sample. Adv Dent Res 1997;11(2): 272–80.

[25] Lamster IB. Oral health care services for older adults: a looming crisis. Am J Public Health 2004;94(5):699–702.

[26] Davenport JC, Basker RM, Heath JR, et al. Need and demand for treatment. Br Dent J 2000; 189(7):364–8.

[27] Matear D, Gudofsky I. Practical issues in delivering geriatric dental care. J Can Dent Assoc 1999;65(5):289–91.

[28] US Department of Health and Human Services. National Institutes of Health. National Institute of Dental and Craniofacial Research. A plan to eliminate craniofacial, oral, and dental health disparities. 2002 (revision). Available at: www.nidcr.nih.gov/Research/HealthDisparities/Reports.htm. Accessed August 2004.

[29] Marcus M, Reifel NM, Nakazono TT. Clinical measures and treatment needs. Adv Dent Res 1997;11(2):263–71.

[30] Centers for Disease Control and Prevention. Division of Oral Health. Oral health for older adults fact sheet. 2003.

[31] Hendricson WD, Cohen PA. Oral health in the 21st century: implications for dental and medical education. Acad Med 2001;76(12):1181–206.

[32] Ajwani S, Tervonen T, Narhi TO, et al. Periodontal health status and treatment needs among the elderly. Spec Care Dentist 2001;21(3):98–103.

[33] Borrell LN, Burt BA, Neighbors HW, et al. Social factors and periodontitis in an older population. Am J Public Health 2004;94(5):748–54.

[34] Lalla E, Park DB, Papapanou PN, et al. Oral disease burden in northern Manhattan patients with diabetes mellitus. Am J Public Health 2004;94(5):755–8.

[35] Brunton PA, Kay EJ. Prevention. Part 6: Prevention in the older dentate patient. Br Dent J 2003;195(5):237–41.

[36] Skrepcinski FB, Jones CM, Reifel N, et al. Indian Health Service. The oral health of adults and elders. IHS Prim Care Provid 2002;27(1):1–5.

[37] Caplan DJ, Hertz-Picciotto I. Racial differences in survival of oral and pharyngeal cancer patients in North Carolina. J Public Health Dent 1998;58(1):36–43.

[38] Drury TF, Garcia I, Adesanya M. Socioeconomic disparities in adult oral health in the United States. Ann NY Acad Sci 1999;896:322–4.

[39] Riley JL, Gilbert GH, Heft MW. Socioeconomic and demographic disparities in symptoms of orofacial pain. J Public Health Dent 2003;63(3):166–73.

[40] Andersen RM, Davidson PL. Ethnicity, aging, and oral health outcomes: a conceptual framework. Adv Dent Res 1997;11(2):203–9.

[41] Strayer MS, Kuthy RA, Caswell RJ, et al. Predictors of dental use of low-income, urban elderly persons upon removal of financial barriers. Gerontologist 1997;37(1):110–6.

[42] Centers for Disease Control and Prevention. At a glance—healthy aging: preventing disease and improving quality of life among older Americans. 2004. Available at: www.cdc.gov/OralHealth/factsheets/adult-order.htm. Accessed July 2004.

[43] McGrath C, Bedi R. Measuring the impact of oral health on quality of life in Britain using OHQoL-UK(W). J Public Health Dent 2003;53(2):73–7.

[44] Centers for Disease Control and Prevention. Health disparities experienced by Hispanics—United States. MMWR Morbid Mortal Wkly Rep 2004;5340:935–7.

[45] Rhee K. US creating a national, transdisciplinary community of clinicians who serve the underserved. J Health Care Poor Underserved 2004;15:1–3.

[46] Formicola AJ, Ro M, Marshall S, et al. Strengthening the oral health safety net: delivery models that improve access to oral health care for uninsured and underserved populations. Am J Public Health 2004;94(5):702–4.

ELSEVIER
SAUNDERS

THE DENTAL
CLINICS
OF NORTH AMERICA

Dent Clin N Am 49 (2005) 377–388

Interaction with Other Health Team Members in Caring for Elderly Patients

Samuel C. Durso, MD

*Division of Geriatric Medicine and Gerontology,
Johns Hopkins University School of Medicine, John R. Burton Pavilion,
5505 Hopkins Bayview Circle, Baltimore, MD 21224, USA*

An 85-year-old retired teacher experiences gradual memory loss over several years. She has hypertension, diabetes mellitus controlled with an oral hypoglycemic drug, and atrial fibrillation for which she takes warfarin to prevent stroke. Two years earlier she underwent successful total hip replacement. After careful medical and functional evaluation, her internist concludes that she is in the early stages of Alzheimer's disease. He is concerned about her ability to live alone and, in particular, to continue to manage her medications safely. Her daughter lives in another city but arranges a consultative visit with the physician to discuss her mother's future care. Because the daughter travels frequently for business, she and her mother decide that an assisted living facility near the daughter's home would provide the safest environment. This plan requires moving to a new city and establishing health care with new providers.

The United States population of adults aged 65 and older is projected to grow from 35 million in 2000 (12.4% of the total population) to 70 million in 2030 (20.6% of the population) [1]. As a result, dentists, physicians, and other health care professionals will care for an ever larger number of individuals living to an advanced old age, many of whom, like the woman described in the vignette, will become frail, suffer multiple chronic illnesses, and experience disability [2].

Furthermore, care of these complex patients occurs in multiple sites and is managed by multiple providers over time. Expert care of geriatric patients often depends on consultation and coordination of services with other professionals and care providers. Consequently, safe and comprehensive care demands teamwork. Understanding the contribution that other health

E-mail address: sdurso@jhmi.edu

team members make to the patient's care and how best to interact with them is an essential competency in geriatrics.

To appreciate the complexity of this challenge, it is helpful to address the following questions:

Who are health care team members?
What information should they collect and share?
How can that information be transmitted effectively to other team members?

Although answers to these questions depend in part on local relationships and resources, a general overview can serve to guide clinicians who are confronted with caring for an older patient.

The health care team

The patient and her daughter choose an assisted living facility owned and operated by a registered nurse who employs two nurse's assistants to care for 12 residents. The facility requires that all residents have a primary care physician, and state law requires that the patient be screened for tuberculosis and undergo a complete medical evaluation, including cognitive and functional assessments. The daughter arranges this evaluation with a local internal medicine group. The initial evaluation is a geriatric assessment performed by a nurse practitioner, which includes a complete physical examination, functional assessment, and coordination of other services based on the patient's needs. The nurse practitioner schedules the patient for a return visit with an internist in the group practice. She also asks the office staff to help the daughter schedule a comprehensive oral health evaluation with a nearby dental group.

Ideally, members of a dental or medical practice work as a team. Each member of the staff performs specific and necessary tasks in a well-coordinated fashion [3]. When the patient has few health problems, as is the case for most young adults, consultation and care coordination with other health care professionals and caregivers are rarely necessary. However, elderly patients, by virtue of disabilities or multiple chronic conditions, are often interacting with nurses, caregivers, and other health care providers simultaneously. As a result, these providers, who are not part of the dentist's or physician's immediate staff, must be included in health care decisions ranging from logistical planning, such as scheduling appointments, to evaluating complex treatment choices. Keeping them informed can be a daunting challenge. Nonetheless, it is vital for the provision of safe and effective care to vulnerable elderly patients.

Who are the members of the health care team? Sometimes the list is extensive. In some instances, clergy and social workers are active contributors. However, the most common participants, in addition to the physician, dentist, and their staff, are informal caregivers (ie, spouse, children, or friends), formal caregivers (ie, registered and licensed practical nurses), and midlevel health care providers (ie, physicians' assistants and nurse practitioners).

Informal caregivers

Because aging so often is associated with increased physical dependency, many older individuals rely on others for assistance with activities of daily living (eg, personal care, including routine oral hygiene) or advanced functions (eg, arranging appointments, adhering to prescriptions). Depending on the patient's residence and health status, this assistance may be provided by informal caregivers (eg, family or friends) or formal caregivers (eg, nurses' aides). In the United States, spouses and children perform by far the greatest part of the care and assistance provided to elderly persons [4]. Although the care-giving role often is viewed as personally rewarding or as a duty, it may impose a significant burden on the caregiver's time and resources. Dentists and physicians should assess a caregiver's burden and watch for signs of fatigue or burn-out (eg, depression, self-neglect, elder abuse).

Patients with cognitive deficits sometimes rely on family or others for assistance with health care decisions. Older persons with mild-to-moderate dementia typically retain their capacity to make personal choices. However, as dementia becomes more advanced, many lose the ability to make difficult decisions (eg, choosing between different treatments). When the need to make difficult decisions arises, patients sometimes turn to informal care-givers for advice or defer to their spouses or children. In most instances, this surrogate decision-making is not delegated through a formal legal process but is stated as a preference by the patient or is implicit in his or her relationship to the caregiver. (An example would be a demented patient who lives with a spouse or child and is unable to make moderately complex decisions.)

When an informal caregiving relationship exists, it is important that the health care provider include the caregiving individual, when appropriate, in a discussion regarding the patient's care. This principle is usually self-evident for extreme dependency but is easily overlooked when the patient is less obviously dependent. For instance, a dentist or physician may not know that the family member or friend is assuming greater responsibility for the executive functions, such as banking or shopping, of an older patient who is well-groomed, socially appropriate, and living alone. Unfortunately, when patients like these are confronted with new information or tasks, they may become confused or forget what they have agreed to do (eg, change a medication dose). It is important, therefore, that health care providers check with caregivers regarding the patient's level of function before implementing patient care plans.

The health care provider should also ascertain the caregiver's ability to assist the patient. For example, a working child who is able to call a parent daily to check on medication compliance may not be able to assist the parent physically with a daily oral care program. In this example, the dental team should work with the child to develop an alternative strategy.

Open-ended questions and nonjudgmental statements are useful for eliciting the caregiver's comprehension of diagnostic and therapeutic plans. One approach is to ask, "Can you tell me your understanding of the plan?" Sometimes a statement of empathy followed by a question is appropriate. For example, "I know that it is difficult to carry out a plan like this. Do you have any concerns?" Caregivers can use this opportunity to provide feedback and discuss barriers. Even straightforward plans (eg, taking an antibiotic three times a day for 1 week) should be reinforced with a brief written instruction provided to the patient or caregiver. A copy should be kept for the patient's dental or medical record.

Long-term care staff

Although most adults over age 65 live independently, more than 1.5 million individuals live in nursing homes, and more than 600,000 individuals live in assisted living facilities. Although the number of nursing home beds has actually declined in the last decade, the number of assisted living facilities and retirement communities is increasing [4].

Individuals in nursing homes and assisted living facilities are generally sicker than in years past, and residents consequently require a high level of personal and medical care. Typically, resident care is provided directly by aides under the supervision of registered or licensed nurses. Nurse administrators provide facility oversight, and physicians spend relatively little time directly overseeing the daily care of long-term care patients.

Although nurses supervise and implement treatment care plans, nursing assistants and aides with various levels of training provide the bulk of personal care to nursing home and assisted living residents. For this reason, aides often are the most reliable resource for assessing the patient's daily care, such as oral hygiene, food intake, and other personal care functions. These important members of the health care team should be considered when trying to ascertain a patient's care needs or when formulating a treatment plan. A telephone call or discussion with the patient's aide during rounds may provide key information or buy-in to a therapeutic plan. The aide's insight into the patient's behaviors and other aspects of the patient's care often proves invaluable, and his or her commitment may be the factor that ensures a care plan's success.

Increasingly, nurse practitioners (also referred to as advanced practice nurses) and physicians' assistants perform day-to-day medical evaluation and management of institutionalized patients. They are also assuming a larger role in ambulatory primary care and specialty practices. Studies indicate that nurse practitioners and physicians' assistants, working as part of a coordinated team with physicians, reduce the hospitalization rates of nursing home residents [5]. Nurse practitioners and, in most states, physicians' assistants can prescribe medication and perform specific procedures under the supervision of a physician. In some states, nurse practitioners are licensed to practice independently. The range of services provided by nurse practitioners and physicians' assistants varies with the practice setting but includes routine and urgent patient visits, home visits, nursing home and assisted living facility visits, primary health screening and counseling, uncomplicated preoperative evaluations, consultative visits (eg, urinary incontinence evaluation, wound care evaluation and management), and follow-up visits after physician evaluation.

Because nurse practitioners and physicians' assistants increasingly perform routine medical care, they may be the providers with the most intimate knowledge of a patient. It has also become more common for midlevel providers to carry their own panel of primary care patients. In these instances, the nurse practitioner or physicians' assistant takes primary responsibility for communicating directly with other professionals (eg, dentists, cardiologists) about medical evaluation, management, and consultation.

Essential health care information

Health care information should be sufficient to provide a clear understanding of the patient's health status and goals. Providing this information is more challenging for older patients, who frequently have altered function and whose health care goals may change with their general health. Furthermore, health care information must generally include a description of the patient's social support, which is needed to coordinate care with multiple providers (eg, time patient care with caregiver availability, plan pre- and postappointment consultation with another specialist) and support diagnostic and therapeutic plans. Therefore, in addition to the usual elements of the history and physical, physicians and dentists should create a patient care database that includes a functional assessment, detailed social history, and description of the patient's general health care goals. Capturing and transmitting this information requires extra effort, but it is well spent. The contents of a consultative request or report depend solely on the clinician's judgment, but both dentists and physicians should consider the functional assessment, social history, and goals in addition to the traditional elements of the history and physical when formulating a recommendation.

The basic elements of the health record for older adults include

Active and past medical illnesses, including major procedures and hospitalizations
A complete list of prescription drugs, over-the-counter medications, and herbal preparations
Adverse drug reactions, specifying the type of reaction (eg, anaphylactic reaction to penicillin, nausea with codeine)
Social history

Functional and cognitive assessment
Advanced care directives
Physical examination
Special studies (eg, laboratory and radiographic tests)

Depending on the nature of the communication and the needs of the patient, the physician or dentist should extract from this database all information that is essential for the other provider to consider when developing a diagnostic or therapeutic plan. Although most items are self-explanatory, the social history, functional and cognitive assessments, and goals of care, including advanced care directives, deserve special mention.

Social history

The social history should provide contact information for formal and informal caregivers and a description of the geriatric patient's living situation (eg, private residence, assisted living or nursing home), living companions, typical activities, driving habits or transportation, personal habits (eg, tobacco and alcohol use), and advanced care directives, if any (eg, Living Will, Durable Power of Attorney for Health Care). Even when older adults live with a companion or spouse, it is useful to ask for the name and contact information of another individual to whom they would turn if they needed help. It also is important for office staff to notice whom, if anyone, the patient wants notified about test results, appointments, or other communications.

Functional assessment

A functional assessment should be included in the health record for all older adults. It should be reviewed initially and updated periodically or after a significant change in health status. The two most common designations of function are activities of daily living (ADL) and instrumental activities of daily living (IADL). ADL include basic functions of self-care (eg, dressing, toileting, transfer, bathing, eating, and grooming, including oral care), whereas IADL designate advanced or executive functions (eg, cooking, driving, bill paying). Usually these activities are designated as independent (I), needs assistance (A), or dependent on others (D).

As adults age, cognitive problems, difficulty with balance, unsafe driving, depression, polypharmacy, bowel changes, and urinary incontinence occur with increasing frequency. Because dentists may be the first point of primary care contact for some older patients, screening questionnaires that include these items may be the best chance for someone with failing health to get early help. Screening for memory loss, often the first sign of dementia, is recommended. An inability to recall three words without error after 1 minute is an indication for further cognitive testing. Falls or driving problems, sadness persisting for more than 2 weeks, changes in bowel habits, troublesome urinary incontinence, excessive alcohol use, and use of sedating medications or dangerous combinations of medications should all be noted. If any of these problems is new or has not been medically evaluated, referral to a primary care provider is indicated. Elder abuse or neglect is unfortunately more common than many health professionals realize. If suspected, it should be reported to the primary physician or other proper authorities.

Decisional support and advanced directives

As with younger patients, there is considerable variation in values and goals among older patients. However, as individuals approach the end of life, their health preferences typically shift from an emphasis on longevity to preserving function, comfort, and dignity. Furthermore, individuals with decisional capacity have the right to make personal choices and the right to change their minds [4]. Consequently, it is important to assess health care goals initially and update them periodically.

When evidence suggests that an older patient needs a higher level of assistance or is a danger to him- or herself or others, the dentist should refer the patient for comprehensive medical and functional assessment.

In many instances, the failing older person retains the capacity to make personal decisions, but he or she or the family needs guidance. Areas of common concern to caregivers include cognitive decline and behavioral abnormalities, inadequate access to food, self-neglect, loneliness produced by social isolation, unsafe driving, depression, alcohol abuse, and need for additional support in ADL. Local departments of aging, Meals on Wheels, and other organizations that address the health and social needs of older adults provide valuable services. Primary care providers should be able to assist dentists and their older patients in accessing these agencies.

Decisional capacity is determined on the basis of a patient's ability to understand the consequences of his or her decision. In most instances, caregivers who have a standing relationship with patients help them with treatment decisions. Their participation in decision making should be noted in the record. When individuals are incapable of making health care decisions, as occurs during advanced stages of Alzheimer's disease, either statutory law determines who has decisional rights regarding a patient's health care (eg, spouse) or this person is designated through a Durable Power of Attorney for Health Care or determined by the presence of a Living Will. Existence of these documents also should be noted in the patient's health record.

Effective communication

The nurse practitioner discovers significant gingivitis and gum recession as part of the patient's nutritional and oral health care screening. She has the patient's daughter make an appointment for an oral examination with a nearby dental group and sends the dentist a consultative request. In it she provides a summary of the patient's medical history and asks that the dentist address specific questions about the patient's oral health and care plan.

In an ideal health system, complete, accurate patient care information would flow to all providers easily and quickly. This efficiency would be a major step in the direction of providing safe care for all patients, especially for those who are old and frail. However, until a system like this becomes commonplace, health care teams (including office staff) must continue to collect accurate, timely patient care information and communicate it to all providers who make patient care decisions. Although the effort may seem burdensome, accurate and timely information increases patient satisfaction, reduces error, and improves office efficiency.

Communication with informal or formal caregivers and nursing staff usually involves a written or telephone communication to discuss a medication change or other therapeutic plan. Verbal medication orders to nursing staff in long-term care facilities are usually transmitted by telephone. A copy of the order is sent to the physician or dentist's office for signature. Telephone conversations and changes in the medication and treatment plan should be documented in the patient's chart [6].

Communication between dentists, physicians, and, increasingly, nurse practitioners and physicians' assistants often involves consultative requests or reports. Telephone calls are appropriate when the information must be obtained quickly, as may occur in an emergency, or the problem is complex and requires discussion.

Sometimes a telephone call is needed for clarification following a written consultation. Medical and dental staff should adopt a policy of notifying dentists and physicians when another professional calls. This policy should include nurse practitioners, physicians' assistants, and licensed nurses performing home health evaluations who are involved in direct patient care and who need to discuss immediate patient care issues. In some cases, providers are traveling from one site of care to another (eg, nursing home, assisted living facility, home visit). As a result, they may need to make a patient care decision or give a caregiver patient care instructions. If the call cannot be taken immediately, the office staff should arrange for the dentist or physician to return the call as soon as possible. In general, a written record of telephone conversations about patient care decisions should be entered into the patient's chart. If the conversation required an important action by one of the parties, then a summary of the conversation should be made and sent to the other party for his or her confirmation.

Written communication, whether as a standard form or letter, should be complete, brief, and legible [7]. Standard forms are convenient and work well for consultative requests or reports of low complexity (eg, low-risk dental procedure in a patient with uncomplicated medical problems). They help ensure that the information recorded is uniform and complete. Most forms, however, have limited space and are not ideal for addressing complex issues. When patients have multiple and complex problems, reports, or requests, a letter, perhaps followed by a telephone call, is the best option.

For straightforward clinical problems, consultative communication usually follows the traditional format in which one professional, usually a dentist or primary care physician, requests service or an opinion of a specialist. Requests for consultation should pose clear, unambiguous questions to the consulting dentist, physician, or other health professional. A clear question should be posed or request for service made followed by a report. Requests that simply state "Please provide a preoperative assessment for patient with heart murmur" are not helpful. In this example, where a patient with a pending dental procedure reports the presence of a heart murmur, the dentists wants to confirm its presence and know whether, in the opinion of the physician, the heart valve abnormality poses a high, moderate, or low risk for bacterial endocarditis. Likewise, consulting dentists and physicians should make their recommendations clear and explicit. For example, if an oral surgeon requests a preoperative assessment of mortality and morbidity risks for a 75-year-old diabetic patient, the physician should state the risk using accepted preoperative assessment tools, such as the Goldman Index [8,9].

Dentists and physicians are responsible for their respective treatment decisions. Therefore, they should consider advice from consultants but should ultimately decide on a plan that is consistent with their best professional judgment. For example, a physician consultant may confirm or deny the presence of a heart murmur and offer an opinion as to the patient's risk for bacterial endocarditis. However, the decision to use prophylactic antibiotics lies primarily with the treating dentist.

In caring for geriatric patients with complex health problems, the consultative communication often goes beyond a simple request for an opinion or service; it becomes a dialogue in which information is exchanged and becomes part of a comprehensive health plan for the patient. Both parties, in effect, are consultants and contribute specific professional expertise. Each offers relevant opinions about those aspects of care for which he or she is responsible and must obtain clarification from the other on how best to proceed (Figs. 1 and 2).

In the same vein, the consultative letter may serve to introduce one provider to another, to establish one's role in the patient's care, to update the patient's health care database, or to educate a colleague about important standards of care in the consultant's area of expertise.

Two aspects of the consultative letter deserve specific comment. As a mechanism for updating the patient's health record and database, consultative letters reduce medical error and limit redundant testing. Second, consultative letters can educate professionals from different disciplines about important practice standards in the consultant's field. For example, many physicians caring for geriatric patients are unaware of the relative benefit and low cardiovascular risks of fractional doses of epinephrine used with local anesthetic, or of the low bleeding risks posed by most dental procedures. A consultative letter from the dentist that explicitly

Date

John Smith, DDS
Address
Telephone number

Re: Jane Doe
Date of Birth

Dear Dr. Smith,

      I recently met and examined Mrs. Jane Doe. She is scheduled to see you on DD/MM/YY for a comprehensive oral assessment.

      In summary, she is a delightful 85 year-old retired schoolteacher who plans to move into the Best Care Assisted Living facility on DD/MM/YY. Her medical problems include gradual functional decline over several years due to memory loss, hypertension, diabetes controlled with oral medication and atrial fibrillation for which she takes warfarin. She underwent successful total hip replacement in 2002. In addition, I noted on oral assessment that she has gingivitis and periodontal disease. I suspect that she has trouble performing oral self-care.

      Currently, she lives with her daughter who assures that she takes her medication. Her daughter will accompany her to your office. We can monitor her anti-coagulation in our office. She is scheduled to see Dr. Mary Jones (internal medicine) in our office on XX/MM/YY to review her medical care plan.

      In your consultative report, I would request that you address the following:
1.   Can your office develop an oral care plan for the assisted living staff?
2.   Does the patient need antibiotic prophylaxis for the hip prosthesis?
3.   Depending on your recommendations, please advise regarding any recommended changes for the anticoagulant and hypoglycemic medications?

      Included is a copy of my initial evaluation, including a list of her medications, and medical care plan. Dr. Jones and I look forward to working with you and your staff to coordinate her medical and dental care. Your staff has our office contact information. Please write or call if I can provide additional information that would be helpful.

Sincerely,

Martha Davis, CRNP

cc: (daughter)

enclosure:

Fig. 1. Example of consultative letter from nurse practitioner to dentist.

addresses these concerns is useful to the physician, nurse practitioner, or physician's assistant in planning medical aspects of the patient's care. It also is helpful when the consulting dentists include citations from dental scientific literature, policies produced by dental and other professional groups, and evidence-based guidelines to support their treatment recommendations.

Date

Martha Davis, CRNP
Address
Telephone number

Re: Mrs. Anyone
Date of Birth

Dear Ms. Davis:

I am writing in regard to our mutual patient, Mrs. Jones. As you know, she has hypertension, diabetes controlled with oral medication and atrial fibrillation for which she takes warfarin. Two years ago she underwent successful total hip replacement. For several years she has experienced gradual memory loss and decreased ability to manage her own affairs. She plans to move into the Best Care Assisted Living facility next month.

Her daughter confirms that she is taking hydrochlorthiazide 25 mg/day, lisinopril 5 mg/day and warfarin 5 mg/day. Our staff also discovered that she takes a non-prescription antihistamine for sleep. She has no history of adverse drug reactions.

My examination revealed gingivitis with extensive gum recession and two root caries. I agree that reduced oral care may be contributing to her periodontal and tooth disease. I also note that she has dry mouth, which may be exacerbated by the non-prescription antihistamine.

I recommend removal of the plaque and calculus and filling the caries. This will be performed over two or three visits. The procedures will require local anesthesia with a small amount of vasoconstrictor. This should not raise her heart rate or blood pressure. Significant bleeding is not expected if her INR is maintained in the therapeutic range. Our staff will schedule the patient to have her INR checked in your office one day prior to the procedures and your staff will fax the results to our office. She may eat and take her hypoglycemic medication before the procedures. She is at low risk for hip prosthesis infection, and therefore I do not recommend antibiotic prophylaxis.

My staff will help the assisted living staff develop an oral care program for the patient. I also recommend stopping the anti-histamine, if you agree.

Please contact our office to confirm the patientís history and antihistamine use. I would also appreciate your recommendations or any concerns you may have about the proposed dental plan.

I will await your reply,

Sincerely,

John Smith, DDS

Fig. 2. Example of consultative letter from dentist to nurse practitioner.

The structure of the consultative note depends on whether it is a request, a response, or some combination of the two. All consultative letters should contain

Patient and caregiver identification and contact information
A brief summary of the history, functional assessment, and social support
All medications and drug reactions

Physicians or dentists requesting consultation should remember that Medicare requires that bills submitted for a consultation identify the individual requesting it. The professional group name is insufficient.

Consultants responding to a request for consultation should address

The specific question being asked
Problem assessment
Proposed procedure, treatment, or management decisions, including the method and type of anesthesia or sedation
The outline of responsibilities (ie, who will do what by when)

Including these elements in the consultative letter provides each member of the health care team with an unambiguous map of the care plan.

Summary

Over the next several decades, dentists, physicians, nurses, and caregivers will be challenged to provide safe, efficient health care to a burgeoning number of older adults with complex needs. Although each profession will contribute a unique set of skills, none will be able to provide comprehensive care in isolation from the others. As a result, interaction among dentists, physicians, and others will rely on effective communication and collaboration. Ultimately, dentists, physicians, and nurses will serve geriatric patients best when working as well-coordinated health care teams.

References

[1] Landefeld SC, Callahan CM, Woolard N. General internal medicine and geriatrics: building a foundation to improve the training of general internists in the care of older adults. Ann Intern Med 2003;139:609–14.

[2] Fried L, Ferrucci L, Darer J, et al. Untangling the concepts of disability, frailty and comorbidity: implications for improved targeting and care. J Gerontol 2004;59:255–63.

[3] Grumbach K, Bodenheimer T. Can health care teams improve primary care practice? JAMA 2004;291(10):1246–51.

[4] Cobbs EL, Duthie EH, Murphy JB, editors. Geriatrics review syllabus: a core curriculum in geriatric medicine. 5th edition. Malden (MA): Blackwell Publishing for the American Geriatrics Society; 2002.

[5] Kane RL, Keckhafer G, Flood S, et al. The effect of evercare on hospital use. J Am Geriatr Soc 2003;51:1427–34.

[6] McNabney MK, Andersen RE, Bennett RG. Nursing documentation of telephone communication with physicians in community nursing homes. J Am Med Dir Assoc 2004;5:180–5.

[7] Valenza JA. Coordination of patient care and consultation between the dentist and physician. Gen Dent 1994;42(1):79–82.

[8] Mangano DT, Goldman L. Preoperative assessment of patients with known or suspected coronary disease. N Engl J Med 1995;333(26):1750.

[9] Goldman M, Caldera D, Southwick FS, et al. Multifactorial index of cardiac risk in non-cardiac surgical procedures. N Engl J Med 1988;148:2120–7.

ELSEVIER
SAUNDERS

Dent Clin N Am 49 (2005) 389–410

THE DENTAL
CLINICS
OF NORTH AMERICA

Cognitive Function, Aging, and Ethical Decisions: Recognizing Change

Janet A. Yellowitz, DMD, MPH

Department of Health Promotion and Policy, Baltimore College of Dental Surgery,
University of Maryland, 666 West Baltimore Street, Room 3E02, Baltimore, MD 21201, USA

As the population ages, dental and other health care providers will be working with more older adults (and their family members) with changing cognitive status than ever before in history. The intent of this article is to review common cognitive changes in older adults that will undoubtedly be seen in dental practices. Knowledge of the common signs and symptoms of age-related cognitive changes provides a basis on which to identify individuals with undiagnosed cognitive changes. This article reviews the relationship between cognitive function, aging, and dementia (specifically, mild cognitive impairment and Alzheimer's disease), the role of the dental team in recognizing these conditions, and issues related to obtaining informed consent from cognitively impaired patients.

Older adults often are identified as the most physically and psychologically heterogeneous adult cohort. Although all organ systems demonstrate some decline with increasing age, each system "ages" at a different rate. Older adults exhibit a wide array of cognitive abilities, ranging from functioning similar to that of younger people to mild impairment to clinical dementia [1,2]. One of the hallmarks of aging is a progressive loss of function, with functionally disabling cognitive declines generally indicating the presence of disease. Because of their enormous impact on individuals, families, the health care system, and society as a whole, cognitive impairments present a major health problem in the United States.

Identifying cognitive abilities can be challenging when working with individuals who have a lifetime of experience and are competent to make decisions [3], particularly because individuals with dementia present with a range of impairments, depending on the disease stage and cause, and a range of abilities (some preserved, some impaired). An increasingly important part of the health care of older adults is identifying their

---

E-mail address: jay001@dental.umaryland.edu

0011-8532/05/$ - see front matter © 2005 Elsevier Inc. All rights reserved.
doi:10.1016/j.cden.2004.10.010   *dental.theclinics.com*

decision-making capacity and preferences for health care. Providing health care to cognitively impaired persons presents a range of ethical dilemmas, with competence a crucial concern. Research into the decision-making competence of cognitively impaired elderly persons is a growing field that is beginning to yield findings with practical implications for preserving the autonomy and welfare of this group of vulnerable patients [4].

The following scenarios are real-life dental office experiences. They are presented as opportunities to identify patients' cognitive changes. Is it possible that these events could occur in your practice? Are you prepared to recognize cognitive changes in older adults?

1. You have just presented a $6000 treatment plan to your patient, a 74-year-old retired college professor. The patient has received extensive dental care throughout his lifetime and has always been prompt for appointments. Although his wife usually accompanies him, she is not with him today, and he says this is because she is not feeling well. Recently, he missed a couple of appointments, despite having been reminded by telephone the previous day. Following a comprehensive examination, you review the treatment plan and its rationale with the patient to obtain consent and authorization for payment. After asking a few questions about using his credit card for payment and the length of time needed to complete the treatment, the patient consents to the care and signs the authorization for payment with his credit card. A series of appointments are scheduled and the patient leaves. Later that day you receive a frantic telephone call from the patient's wife, seeking an explanation for the $6000 credit card charge for her husband's "teeth cleaning"—or, at least, that is what her husband told her he received at your office. When asked why the bill is so high, he claims to be unsure but suggests that it was a mistake and there is no need to worry about it.

2. While waiting to talk with the dentist following a routine visit with the dental hygienist, a 67-year-old female patient talks about how proud she is of her three grandchildren. The practice and the dental hygienist have known the patient for many years. Early in the appointment, the hygienist noticed that the patient appeared out of sorts and distracted. When questioned, the patient said that it was nothing; she had just been rushing around and was almost late for the appointment. The hygienist becomes even more concerned about the patient when she is unable correctly to name her three grandchildren, who live down the street from her. Instead of naming her grandchildren, the patient identifies her two children and says the name of the third is on the "tip of her tongue." They laugh, and the hygienist says that she understands: things like this happen all the time. After the appointment, the dental hygienist again asks the patient whether she remembers the name of her third grandchild. The patient appears a bit confused by the question; she then identifies two grandchildren but still cannot remember the third name.

3. You are asked to see an emergency patient by a colleague. The patient is an 85-year-old gentleman complaining of chronic left-sided facial pain. He is unsure how long the pain has been present; however, it is fairly uncomfortable at the moment. The patient is married but has come to the appointment alone. The patient presents a list of 13 medications but is unclear about when or why he takes them. The clinician recommends that the patient keep cold compresses on his face for 20 minutes every hour and return the following day with his medication bottles and his wife. The dentist is unsure the patient will remember the instructions and is unsure how to proceed.

These cases exemplify some of the intricacies of identifying possible cognitive changes in older adult patients. Have you experienced one of these situations or something similar? Are these patients demented, delirious, or "just old"? To help reduce the chances that these or similar situations will occur, this article provides dentists with information to improve their skills in detecting cognitive changes in their patients. The last section of the article provides a list of suggestions for avoiding and/or managing these situations.

Memory and aging: is it normal to lose cognitive function with age?

People have always lived to extreme old age without severe memory loss, although memory loss has been attributed to the aging process [5]. Changes in brain structure and function are inevitable age-related events. For example, some neurons shrink, neurofibrillary tangles develop, and beta-amyloid plaques develop around neurons. In addition, there is free radical damage and an increase in inflammation. Although these events are ongoing, longitudinal studies have demonstrated that many, if not most, older adults maintain their cognitive function throughout their lifetimes.

Memory changes are the most common cognitive complaints reported by older adults. Yet many memory processes do not appear to change with successful aging, and an older adult's memory is typically adequate for the demands of independent living. Remote memory (recall of events that occurred in the distant past), sensory memory, and semantic memory (ie, vocabulary and general information about the world) remain largely unchanged in older adults. Verbal abilities also remain stable with normal aging. In contrast, nonverbal creative thinking and new problem-solving strategies show a slow decline with age [6].

Many factors influence memory and cognitive ability in older adults. Relevance and time of day influence functional abilities. Hess et al [7] found that older adults' memory and decision accuracy improve when they perceive the task to be personally relevant or are held accountable for their performances. Others have found that when older adults are given materials that engage their emotional interest, their performance on memory tests equals that of young adults [8]. Time of day also has been identified as a factor in memory, with older adults performing better at their optimal time of day on most memory tasks. This time is determined by a biologic clock that appears to shift toward the morning as a person ages [9].

Horn and Cattell [10] suggest that crystallized abilities (information and skills gained from experience) remain relatively intact with aging, whereas fluid intelligence, which involves flexible reasoning and problem solving, declines. Attention, namely the ability to focus on one or more pieces of visual or auditory information long enough to register and make meaningful use of the data, does not change with aging. However, one's attention can be altered by perceptual or sensory changes, illness, chronic pain, medications, and psychologic disturbance (in particular, depression and anxiety)—all common in older adult populations.

The most common reasons for acute confusional states in elderly patients are adverse drug events and drug interactions. Medications are the most common cause of acutely reversible cognitive impairment, which is often due to declines in homeostatic processes, such as drug absorption, distribution, metabolism, and excretion change [11]. Drug absorption and metabolism are further affected by age-associated decreases in stomach acidity, splanchnic blood flow, peristalsis, and stomach emptying time.

Because of the presence of comorbid medical conditions, the use of medications taken for central nervous system effects (eg, benzodiazepines, neuroleptics, antihistamines) and the use of over-the-counter medications make it crucial for health care providers to review all medications with patients before prescribing additional ones, and when the provider is suspicious of a cognitive change. Other significant common causes of dementia in the elderly are dehydration, fluid or electrolyte derangement, pain, and infection.

Cognitive impairments and aging—what is dementia?

Dementia is a generic term used to designate chronically progressive brain disease that impairs intellect and behavior to the point where customary activities of daily living become compromised [12]. The word comes from two Latin words that translate as "away" and "mind." It is not the name of a specific disease but rather a description of a clinical state and does not imply causation or prognosis.

Dementia is a global impairment of the intellect, memory, and personality without alteration of consciousness. It has been characterized as acting confused, talking or mumbling to oneself, repeating the same thing over and over, hearing or seeing things that are not there, forgetting the names of family members or close friends, forgetting the right words to use, yelling or swearing at people, interfering or offering unwanted advice, acting restless or agitated, acting fearful without good reason, complaining or criticizing, showing inappropriate sexual behavior, wandering outside the house, and refusing to be left alone.

In the past, dementia was designated by many names, including hardening of the arteries, senility, and organic brain syndrome. Dementia, as described by the American Psychiatric Association in its *Diagnostic and Statistical Manual of Mental Disorders* [13], is the development of multiple cognitive deficits that include memory impairment and at least one of the following:

- Aphasia (deterioration of language function)
- Apraxia (impaired ability to execute motor activities, despite intact motor abilities, sensory function, and comprehension of the task)
- Agnosia (failure to recognize or identify objects despite sensory function)
- Disturbance in executive functioning (ie, ability to think in abstractions and to plan, initiate, sequence, monitor, and stop complex behavior)

In addition, the cognitive deficits must be sufficiently severe to cause impairment in occupational or social functioning, such as working, shopping, dressing, bathing, or handling finances, and they must represent a decline from a previous level of functioning [13]. As the disease progresses, those with dementia become impaired in their ability to learn new material and forget previously learned material. Victims may lose valuables like wallets and keys, forget food cooking on the stove, or become lost in familiar neighborhoods.

Persons with dementia exhibit numerous specific changes in cognitive performance. The abilities commonly affected in dementia include verbal and nonverbal memory, perceptual-organizational abilities, communication skills, and psychomotor performance. The early signs of dementia often are subtle and can easily be passed off as a normal reaction to emotional upset or other physical ailments. Short-term memory loss is usually the first recognizable sign of a developing problem. Although the person is able to reminisce about significant past events in great detail, he or she may start to forget the names of close friends and family, miss appointments, or repeat certain tasks over and over. Balancing a checkbook or counting change can become problematic. The individual may become confused and restless. Often people with dementia experience disorientation to time and place, or they may start to withdraw from the daily activities of life and show a general apathy marked by unusual outbursts of aggressiveness, hyper-sexuality, and irritability.

Many reversible and irreversible conditions can mimic dementia in older adults, making the prognosis of dementia dependent on the underlying cause. Alzheimer's disease is the most common cause of dementia in older adults, but cognitive deficits may have many causes, including degenerative central nervous system conditions that cause progressive deficits in memory or cognition (eg, Parkinson's disease, Huntington's disease, amyotrophic lateral sclerosis or multiple sclerosis), systemic conditions (eg, hypothyroid-ism, vitamin B12 deficiency, HIV infection), structural brain damage (hemorrhagic or occlusive cerebrovascular disease, normal pressure hydrocephalus, meningioma or subdural hematoma), and substance abuse (eg, alcohol). Infections such as cerebral, fungal, and parasitic infections and tertiary stage syphilis (usually 15 to 30 years after acute exposure) can mimic dementia. As many as two thirds of individuals with AIDS have AIDS-related cognitive changes, but these changes are the sole presenting symptom in less than 10% of HIV-infected individuals. In many patients with dementia, no underlying cause is identified.

Wide variation is seen from person to person in rates of decline and in the rapidity with which the dementing process progresses [14]. The nature, extent, and rate of decline depend on the underlying cause, the person's educational level, and the person's general health status. Depending on the type and stage of disease, individuals with dementia may [13]

- Exhibit little or no awareness of memory loss or other cognitive abnormalities
- Be spatially disoriented and have difficulty with spatial tasks
- Make unrealistic assessments of their abilities and make plans that are not congruent with their deficits and prognosis (eg, accepting an expensive treatment plan when indigent)
- Underestimate the risks involved in activities (eg, driving)
- Exhibit violent behavior
- Attempt suicide, particularly at early stages when the individual is more capable of carrying out a plan of action
- Have disturbances in their gait, leading to falls
- Show disinhibited behavior, such as making inappropriate jokes or comments, neglecting personal hygiene, exhibiting undue familiarity with strangers, or disregarding conventional rules of social conduct
- Have delusions, especially ones involving themes of persecution (eg, the belief that misplaced possessions have been stolen)
- Be vulnerable to physical stressors (eg, illness or minor surgery) and psychosocial stressors (eg, going to the dental office or hospital or through bereavement)

Prospective studies of subjects with clinically evident dementia show that subtle symptoms often occur many years before the dementia can be diagnosed.

Early in the disease process, there often is a growing awareness that something is wrong. Both the person with dementia and those closest to them may be aware of the changes and concerned about how best to address memory lapses, functional impairments, or periods of confusion. Because dementia-like behaviors can have a large number of reversible causes, it is crucial to identify the cause of the behavior as soon as possible. Unrecognized cognitive impairments may lead to iatrogenic illness, unnecessary work-ups driven by vague symptoms, inappropriate and costly use of health care, and poor outcomes. Early and accurate diagnosis of these conditions gives patients a greater chance to benefit from existing treatments and allows them and their families to plan for the future. Because this early phase may last for years, it is important for family and caregivers to monitor the individual's behavior over time.

Recognizing cognitive changes in older adults: the role of oral health professionals

Assessing cognitive changes in older adults can be challenging to the professional, because they often retain their social skills and ability to make customary social remarks longer than their insight and judgment. Patients may sound fine and appear to respond appropriately but in fact be unable to care for themselves responsibly. Clinicians usually assess cognitive skills intuitively; however, retaining a patient's informal personal information (eg, names of children and grandchildren, hobbies) can be a useful aide in reviewing the patient's memory and checking for cognitive changes. When suspicious, the clinician may ask the patient to describe a typical day, to describe how he or she spends leisure time, or, when applicable, to identify the names of his or her children or grandchildren. These tasks require recall of categories of activities and abstract thinking, which are cognitive abilities that decline early in dementia. The responses must then be corroborated with the patient's caregiver or others knowledgeable of the specific information requested. Like anyone with symptoms of a disease, people with dementia have good days and bad days. Mace et al [15] compared a demented individual's tendency to be able to do something one day and not the next to a loose light bulb that sometimes connects and sometimes fails to connect.

Health care professionals and caregivers often mistake early signs and symptoms of dementia for normal aging changes, thereby perpetuating myths and fallacies about aging and dementia—in particular, the notions that the early signs of dementia are "just old age" or "just senility" or are due to chronic illness. Because early signs and symptoms of dementia are often subtle and nonspecific, clinicians may overlook apparently healthy adults with cognitive impairments [16]. During an office visit, cognitively impaired patients may appear to present appropriately, especially when limited time is spent observing or conversing with them. Dental practitioners may notice memory lapses, missed appointments, symptomatic complaints discordant with clinical evaluation, hearing acuity problems, or deference to a spouse or caregiver in responding to questions, making expensive purchases, or agreeing to an extensive treatment plan.

The low rates of recognition of dementia among health care professionals constitute a major barrier to appropriate care for these patients [17]. Rates of "failure to recognize" have been reported as high as 97% for mild dementia and 50% for moderate dementia [18]. Often these impairments are not recognized until the cognitive loss has become severe. As in the case of other chronic and debilitating diseases, such as cancer and diabetes, the presence of cognitive decline in the dental practice affects the delivery of care. Dental professionals need to be aware of the impact of aging and disease when a patient presents with subtle changes in his or her mental status. Dental care providers are responsible for identifying patients' signs and symptoms of disease to recognize and prevent problems associated with their management and for using consultations and referrals appropriately [19]. It is important for dental professionals to screen and assess the cognitive abilities of older adults and to ensure acceptance of proposed treatment options before proceeding with treatment.

Once patients have been identified as having a problem with memory or with the ability to think clearly, the dental team needs to follow up on these concerns with the patient and his or her caregiver or family member. The dental team can help ensure that the individual and family have a realistic understanding of the illness and its impact on the individual's general and oral health. Likewise, the dental team is responsible for identifying a realistic treatment plan for the individual, taking into account the potential impact of the disease on the individual's oral health behaviors. The dental office may also assist the family in identifying local resources and referrals.

Following a diagnosis of dementia, noticeable changes in mental functioning may be noted in both the diagnosed individual and the caregiver. These reactions include depression, denial, anxiety and fear, isolation and loneliness, embarrassment, shame, and feelings of loss. As the disease progresses, individuals with dementia may experience difficulty performing daily routines, as well as frustration due to their need for assistance with activities of daily living and self-care. Hence the dental team may want to reinforce the need for increased frequency of personal and professional oral health maintenance and routine care.

When dealing with people with dementia and their caregivers, health care professionals should acknowledge their feelings and encourage them to take care of their physical and mental health. Caregivers need to be supported in maximizing their caregiving roles while maintaining an appropriate balance in their personal life. Family roles change as the caregiving system is organized and caregivers take greater control over the impaired elder's life. As dementia progresses, the individual can change from a competent, independent adult into a person who requires help with all activities of daily living.

Mild cognitive impairment

The term "benign senescent forgetfulness" was introduced in 1962 to distinguish individuals with mild, minimally progressive cognitive impairment from those with more malignant progressive dementia [20,21]. In 1990, "mild cognitive impairment" (MCI) was first used to describe individuals with cognitive impairment on neuropsychologic testing who do not meet criteria for dementia and whose impairment is not the result of a known medical condition [22–24]. MCI has also been referred to as age-associated memory impairment and has been identified as a likely early clinical manifestation of Alzheimer's disease [25].

MCI is a clinical entity characterized by recent memory loss greater than expected with normal aging, without significant dysfunction in other cognitive domains or impairment in day-to-day functions (activities of daily living) [26]. Individuals with MCI may present with disturbances in any of the following cognitive functions [13]:

- Memory (learning or recalling new information)
- Executive function (planning, reasoning)
- Attention or speed of information processing (concentration, rapidity of assimilating or analyzing information)
- Perceptual motor abilities (integrating visual, tactile, or auditory information with motor activities)
- Language (eg, word-finding difficulties, reduced fluency)

Although the specifics of MCI are not well defined, there is conceptual agreement that MCI describes older people whose memory or other cognitive abilities are not at the same level as when they were younger. The early cognitive deficits of MCI are usually not significant enough to interfere markedly with daily cognitive and functional activities. The diagnosis of MCI is difficult, because it is dependent on cognitive performance tests, which are subject to practice effects and random variability [5,23,27], as well as on the testing of logical memory, visual reproductions, cognitive flexibility, and other factors [28].

The reported prevalence of MCI varies widely and is dependent on the criteria used. Data on the incidence of MCI are limited, with most published studies having participants from clinics that specialize in memory problems or too few subjects to draw definitive conclusions [5]. The Indianapolis Health and Aging Study reported an overall prevalence of approximately 25% for cognitive impairment without dementia among older persons and found that the incidence of MCI increased with age [29]. The Canadian Health and Aging Study reported 15% of older people as having MCI [28,30] and found that 10% to 15% of patients with MCI converted to dementia each year, totaling 48% in 4 years.

Lyketsos et al [31] found that, like most people with dementia, 43% of those diagnosed with MCI experience neuropsychiatric symptoms, such as depression, apathy, and irritability. In addition, following a diagnosis of MCI, victims often demonstrate a decline on measures of activities of daily living, such as managing financial affairs [32]. MCI victims are two to three times more likely to be placed in a long-term care facility [2,33] and twice as likely to die over the next several years than people without cognitive impairment [33,34].

Longitudinal research suggests that 80% of those diagnosed with MCI will go on to develop Alzheimer's disease within 5 to 8 years, converting at a rate of approximately 10% to 15% per year, as compared with 1% to 2% in the general population [28]. Overall, the risk of Alzheimer's disease appears to be increased between three and eightfold [23,33]. Given the risk of MCI's conversion to dementia, it needs to be identified and treated early, increasing the responsibility of the dental team to identify suspicious findings and to refer patients for comprehensive evaluation.

Alzheimer's disease defined

Alzheimer's disease (AD), or dementia of the Alzheimer's type, the single most common cause of dementia, is an irreversible, chronic disorder with a gradual onset and a slowly progressive course that is characterized by an inevitable deterioration in cognitive function [35]. Although memory loss is a feature of all dementias, the cardinal feature of AD is a progressive loss of memory of recent events and experiences. AD affects every individual differently, and there is no way to determine precisely how the disease will present and progress. Although the disease has no cure, some of its symptoms can be treated with medications and behavioral approaches.

AD was first described by Alois Alzheimer in 1906. The pathognomonic beta amyloid extracellular neuritic plaques and intracellular neurofibrillary tangles, which Alzheimer first observed, continue to be necessary for postmortem confirmation [14]. It is believed that the clinical symptoms of AD are preceded by a period of unknown duration (years to decades) during which neuropathologic alterations accumulate in the AD brain without detectable changes in cognition [14,25].

The greatest risk factor for AD is increasing age (generally ≥ 60 years), although it has been found in much younger individuals. Excluding persons with clinically questionable dementia, AD has a prevalence of approximately 1% among those aged 65 to 69 years, which increases to 40% to 50% among persons aged 95 years and older [36,37]. In 2003, 4.5 million Americans were estimated to have AD, twice as many as in 1980 [38]. As the population ages, the disease affects a greater percentage of Americans. Assuming that the number of older adults continues to increase without advances in the prevention or treatment of AD, the number of individuals with AD is expected to grow by 25% over the next 20 years and will range from 11.3 million to 16 million in 2050 [38].

AD constitutes about two thirds of cases of dementia overall (various studies range from 42% to 81%), with vascular causes and other neurodegenerative diseases, such as Pick's disease and diffuse Lewy body dementia, making up most of the remaining cases [36,39]. The prevalence of AD is increased in individuals with Down's syndrome and in individuals with a history of head trauma [13].

Because of cognitive reserve and the subtlety of the pathologic changes, it is difficult to date the onset of the dementia. This reserve may help explain why certain factors (ie, higher education, maintenance of active brain activity) [40] are negative risk factors for the condition. As damage evolves, the reserve is exhausted and the beginnings of impairment become evident. Unfortunately, the clinical diagnosis typically is not made until significant damage has occurred. The overwhelming majority of AD cases are sporadic and nonfamilial and thus are not related to specific genetic mutations.

Dementia is democratic—it knows no social, racial, gender, or economic lines. Typically, memory complaints appear first, although behavioral changes, such as social withdrawal and clustering of affective symptoms, can be the first indications of an important change in the individual's cognitive state [41]. Problems with judgment, problem solving, executive function, planning, and abstract thought are also common in early AD. Behavioral symptoms (noncognitive) are an important but often neglected problem in AD. They create more stress on caregivers than does the cognitive dysfunction itself [42]. Personality changes may range from progressive passivity to marked hostility and can develop before the cognitive impairments. Patients can show decreased emotional expression, increased stubbornness, diminished initiative, and greater suspiciousness [43]. These behavioral changes may be noted in the dental office in an individual presenting with new or worsened procrastination, poor planning, impaired problem solving, or difficulty in handling paperwork (completing health history forms, writing checks, or completing insurance documents).

AD tends to present with an insidious onset, with early deficits in recent memory followed by the development of aphasia, apraxia, and agnosia after several years. In later stages, individuals may develop gait and motor disturbances and eventually may become mute and bedridden. The usual progression of decline is from higher levels of intellectual activities, such as money management, shopping, cooking, reading, and driving, to lower-level activities, such as personal hygiene. Dementia affects the ability to carry out the requisite tasks and contributes to functional decline. Independent living requires the accomplishment of both activities of daily living (ADL), which include self-care tasks such as bathing, grooming, and toileting, and instrumental activities of daily living (IADL), which are cognitively more complex activities such as driving and meal preparation [21–25]. The severity of disease progression in dementia can be demonstrated by performance decline on IADL and ADL tasks. IADL performance decline has been associated with 1-year risk of incident dementia [44].

The average duration from onset of symptoms to death is 8 to 10 years. From the time of diagnosis, people with AD survive about half as long as those of similar age without dementia. Average survival time is affected by age at diagnosis and severity of other medical conditions [45].

Patients with AD come to medical attention because of forgetfulness, usually accompanied by apathy. Apathy, or the lack of motivation or behavioral initiation, is a pervasive problem throughout the course of AD and is perhaps the most common adverse behavior in the illness. Apathetic behaviors are often misattributed to insensitivity, disinterest, and voluntary

---

Box 1. Modification of the Alzheimer's Association's 10 Warning Signs, including examples that may be observed by an oral health care provider or staff members

Memory loss

Forgetting recently learned information is one of the most common early signs of dementia. Although it is normal to forget appointments, names, or telephone numbers, those with dementia forget these things more often and do not remember them later. Patients with memory loss may

- Be more repetitive; ask the same thing over and over, for example, "Are you almost done? Are you almost done? Are you almost done?"
- Forget recent conversations, names, telephone numbers, events, and appointments; misplace objects; come to an appointment at the wrong time or date
- Be poor historians—when unsure, they will "make up" an answer
- Have difficulty discussing current events in an area of interest
- Be unable to remember forgotten thoughts at a later date
- Appear more passive and less responsive; be more irritable and suspicious than usual; misinterpret visual or auditory stimuli
- Repeatedly and apparently unintentionally fail to follow directions; for example, be unable to locate the restroom, even though directions have been provided several times in the past 10 minutes

Difficulty performing familiar tasks—managing routine chores

- Patients may have trouble following a train of thought or performing tasks that require multiple steps, such as following directions to modify a current toothbrush regimen.
- Patients may forget medications or have difficulty taking medications according to instructions.
- Patients may have unexplained weight loss or gain.
- Patients may have difficulty adapting to stressful experiences (eg, death or illness of a spouse, being hospitalized).

Problems with language—word-finding difficulty

Patients may have difficulty finding the words to express what they want to say; for example, when unable to find the toothbrush, patient may ask for "that thing for my mouth."

Disorientation to time and place

It is normal to forget the day of the week or where you are going, but only temporarily. These patients may

- Get lost on their own street or within the confines of a familiar setting
- Organize objects around the house, finding their way around familiar places
- Forget where they are, how they got there, and how to return home

Poor or decreased judgment
No one has perfect judgment all the time. However, these patients may exhibit
- Impaired reasoning ability; inability to respond with a reasonable plan to problems, such as what to do if a fire occurs
- Uncharacteristic disregard for rules of social conduct—for example, loud and negative comments about another person
- Inappropriate clothing and inattention to appearance; difficulty dressing for the weather; may wear several shirts or blouses on a warm day, very little clothing in cold weather, or soiled clothing
- Tendency to give away large amounts of money or pay for unnecessary services

Problems with abstract thinking
Patients may have difficulty writing a check or balancing a checkbook; they may forget what the numbers are and what needs to be done with them.

Misplacing things
Anyone can temporarily misplace a wallet or keys. These patients may put things in unusual places, for example, eyeglasses in the freezer, a wristwatch in the sugar bowl, or a toothbrush in a shoe.

Changes in mood or behavior
Everyone can become sad or moody from time to time. These patients may
- Appear more passive and less responsive; appear uninterested in surroundings
- Show rapid mood swings—from calm to tears to anger—for no apparent reason
- Misinterpret visual or auditory stimuli—for example, be frightened by the sound of a high speed handpiece or want to answer the telephone in your office

Changes in personality
- Patients may become extremely confused, suspicious, fearful, or dependent.

- Patients may defer to a caregiver to answer questions directed to them.

Loss of initiative
- Patients may appear unable to adapt to a new environment, for example, to a new or different office.
- Patients may experience functional difficulties under stress; for example, pain, an emergency, or death or illness of a spouse may precipitate a "bladder accident."
- Patients may become very passive, not wanting to do their usual activities; they may sleep more than usual.

or willful refusal to cooperate on the part of the patient [46]. Misplacing personal objects, repeating questions, and forgetting recent events are among the presenting symptoms. Although the patient may forget people's names, word-finding during conversation is usually not a major problem [12]. In the early stages, passivity and withdrawal are seen in up to two thirds of patients with mild AD [47]. Passive personality change has been identified as predating cognitive abnormality but is only discerned retrospectively. One retrospective review suggested that social withdrawal, mood changes, or depression were present in more than 70% of cases, with a mean duration of more than 2 years before diagnosis of AD [41]. Many with AD do not recognize that they are impaired, an attitude that has been linked to the difficulty in implicit learning of intellectual limitations, rather than to a "denial" of their illness [48].

The recommended criteria for diagnosing AD include

- Insidious onset
- Progressive course
- Memory loss
- At least one other focal cognitive disturbance, such as language dysfunction, apraxia, or executive dysfunction

These impairments should represent a decline from past levels of performance and interfere with established patterns of daily function. Motor functions generally remain normal.

The diagnosis of AD is based largely on clinical findings and can be made only when other causes for the dementia have been excluded. In most AD cases, CT or MRI will reveal brain atrophy, with wider cortical sulci and larger cerebral ventricles than would be expected in the normal aging process. The diagnosis of AD is confirmed only with a postmortem microscopic examination of the brain, which will reveal histopathologic changes, including senile plaques, neurofibrillary tangles, granulovascular degeneration, neuronal loss, and amyloid angiopathy. Minor pathologic changes may appear decades before clinical symptoms occur, and they may also be found in middle-aged and elderly persons without obvious symptoms of the disorder [35].

Individuals with undiagnosed dementia may exhibit behaviors or symptoms that offer a clue to the presence of dementia and can be observed by the dental team. If the individual has increased difficulty with any of the activities listed in the next paragraph, he or she should be referred for a comprehensive assessment to rule out possible causes of disease.

The following list is the Alzheimer's Association 10 Warning Signs. See Box 1 for examples of items on this list that may be observed by an oral health care provider or staff members [49].

Memory loss
Difficulty performing familiar tasks—managing routine chores
Problems with language—word-finding difficulty
Disorientation to time and place
Poor or decreased judgment
Problems with abstract thinking
Misplacing things
Changes in mood or behavior
Changes in personality
Loss of initiative

Once they have identified a patient who has problems with memory or the ability to think clearly, clinicians need to follow up on these concerns with the patient's caregiver or family member. When discussing observations of a patient's cognitive changes with family members, they should emphasize that they have identified a change in behavior and that they are not diagnosing a disease but are suggesting the need for a comprehensive evaluation to identify the cause of this change.

Informed consent: working with the cognitively impaired

Providing oral health care for cognitively impaired older persons presents a range of ethical dilemmas, some of which are addressed in the American Dental Association's (ADA) Principles of Ethics and Code of Professional Conduct. The ADA's Principles of Ethics states that dentists have several affirmative duties toward patients. The ethical principle of beneficence included in the code means that professionals have a duty to act for the benefit of others, "with due consideration being given to the needs, desires and values of the patient." In addition, the principle of autonomy guides dentists in working with impaired patients. This principle states that professionals have a duty to treat the patient according to the patient's desires, within the bounds of accepted treatment, and to protect the patient's confidentiality. Patients with the capacity to make health care decisions should have the right to make decisions about their own bodies, whether or not those decisions are approved by their physicians and families. Because of the impact on treatment planning and overall care, it is important to identify patients' cognitive impairments before obtaining consent and initiating treatment. Unless patients give evidence to the contrary, they are generally presumed capable of deciding about treatment.

Discerning a patient's capacity to consent to treatment can be one of the most challenging aspects of the consent process, given that the ability of patients to make informed decisions can be compromised by illness, medication, or cognitive impairments and that a loss of decision-making capacity (or competency) is an inevitable consequence of dementia. Ensuring that an appropriate consent has been given can be particularly difficult when a patient demonstrates behaviors that reflect a cognitive change but has not been diagnosed with a cognitive impairment. When they are concerned about an individual's decision-making ability, whether because the individual has undergone an abrupt change in mental status, has refused recommended treatment, has consented too hastily to treatment, or is suspicious in other ways for cognitive impairment [50], health care providers should consult with the individual's caregiver, spouse, family member, or primary care physician to discuss his or her decision-making capacity and should refer for evaluation as necessary [51], keeping in mind that these individuals may not be aware of or willing to acknowledge cognitive changes. In general, a physician's confirmation of a patient's cognitive abilities is best following a comprehensive assessment of the patient.

The process of informed consent is the primary mechanism for protecting patient autonomy in treatment decisions [52] and is essential to the delivery of clinical care. The standard for legally competent understanding assumes that the individual can comprehend diagnostic and treatment information. In general, for the informed consent to be valid [53], (1) the patient must be informed; (2) the patient must have free choice; and (3) the patient must have the capacity to consent to treatment.

Although legal standards vary by jurisdiction, four specific abilities need to be addressed when assessing a patient's decision-making capacity, including

The ability to understand information about treatment
The ability to appreciate how that information applies to one's own situation
The ability to reason with that information
The ability to make a choice and express it [50,51]

Based on this information, the practitioner will be better able to evaluate the patient's competency. Assessments of the patient's understanding of treatment options should focus on a specific choice, whereas assessment of the patient's appreciation of the meaning of diagnostic and treatment information should focus on whether the patient can describe the implications of the treatment options [54]. Although they are not addressing the legal concerns of informed consent, practitioners who are developing a treatment plan for a cognitively impaired patient without advance directives may try to identify the patient's prior choice while competent or attempt to identify his or her best interest, in lieu of waiting for a guardianship to be established [55].

Feinberg and others have found that persons with dementia possess sufficient capacity to state specific preferences, make care-related decisions [54,56,57], and be involved in decisions about daily living [55]. Because adults with mild dementia often participate in medical decision making as defined by legal standards, health care professionals need to ensure that these individuals are able to act independently. Most health care providers assess their patients' decision-making capacity within the health care system, but evaluations of decisional capacity made on the basis of a clinical interview are often unreliable [54,58].

Advance health care directives: living wills, health care proxies, power of attorney

Before they become incapacitated to make health care decisions, individuals are advised to prepare documents that direct the provision of their health care when they are no longer able to do so. These documents help health care providers to manage the individual's care as he or she had desired and do not require a consensus answer. To complete these documents, individuals must be 18 years of age and of sound mind; depending on the state, the documents may need to be signed by a witness or notary public. Although all states recognize advance health care directives, each state has its own laws regarding these documents. The first document is a written statement or declaration that details the type of care desired (or not desired) and requires health care personnel to follow these directions. The second document, called a "durable power of attorney for health care," appoints someone to be an individual's health care agent or proxy. In some states, these documents are combined into a single form. Health care directives are also referred to as advance directives, medical directives, directives to physicians, declaration directives, declarations regarding health care, designations of health care surrogate, patient advocate designations, and living wills.

When enacted, the health care proxy grants authority to a second person to make health care decisions for a first person when he or she is unable to express a preference. Generally, this occurs when individuals are unconscious or no longer have the legal capacity to make their own decisions. Physicians are responsible for making the determination regarding an individual's capacity to make his or her own medical treatment decisions, and each state has its own rules and regulations regarding their format and use.

Depending on state law, living wills permit individuals to express their desire to be given life-sustaining treatments in the event of terminal illness or injury and provide other medical directions that affect the end of life. Living wills are thus rarely applicable to the dental environment, but having this information available can be considered good practice on the part of a dental practitioner. In all states, physicians (usually two) determine whether an individual's medical condition warrants the use of a living will.

To say that individuals lack capacity usually means that they cannot understand the nature and consequences of the health care choices presented to them and that they are unable to communicate their own wishes for care, either orally, in writing, or through gestures. Through the use of advance directives, some patients will have their health care concerns addressed before becoming incapacitated. It is crucial for the dental professional to review the documents and verify the extent of the care before initiating treatment.

Clinical judgments about consent capacity are challenging and at times unreliable, especially in older adults who have neurologic conditions with subtle cognitive changes. No standardized instruments to assess competency currently exist, and until a valid and reliable method is devised for this purpose, it behooves clinicians to take whatever measures necessary to ensure the accuracy of their assessment of their patients' cognitive skills.

Summary

With the incidence and prevalence of all dementias increasing along with the longevity and age of the population, the early identification of these ailments is crucial to reducing their associated morbidity and mortality. However, the assessment of cognitive impairments in older adults is complicated by the loss of physiologic reserve, the presence of multiple and chronic diseases, polypharmacy, and the attitude of health care professionals. Although "determining the capacity to make decisions is an inexact science," Wetle [59] suggests that more knowledge and a higher level of suspicion will enable dental professionals better to identify and refer individuals with suspicious cognitive changes. Advances in diagnostic testing and the trend toward earlier diagnosis give health care professionals a greater opportunity for early and consistent involvement in everyday care decisions regarding the person with a cognitive impairment.

Addressing the scenarios: helpful hints and suggestions

Addressing the problems posed at the beginning of this article in an appropriate manner may require spending additional time with each patient. Although many practitioners prefer not to know the personal sides of their patients, one member of the team might be designated to inquire about the patient's life and lifestyle.

Having a dental team familiar with the signs and symptoms of common cognitive changes in older adults reduces the risk of not recognizing patients with cognitive changes. Staff members need to be knowledgeable and empowered to address these concerns with the dentist.

The following is a list of ways in which dental professionals might respond more positively to the given scenarios:

  Receptionist or staff members could question the patient about missed appointments, wife's absence, or illness.

  When reviewing the medical history—when was the last medical visit? were medications added or eliminated?—the practitioner should note changes in medications and patterns of medication use and should ask about medications protocol. He or she should determine the date of the last comprehensive medical evaluation and confirm it with the physician's office if the patient is uncertain.

  Maintaining "social notes" on an individual's chart facilitates conversation and comparisons. Social notes can include names of children and grandchildren, regular vacation spot, family pets, hobbies, and so on. Keep in mind that individuals who have numerous grandchildren with whom they are not in close contact may be unable to identify them all. However, in smaller and more closely knit families, the names of all grandchildren "should" be readily accessible.

  Practitioners should contact a spouse or physician regarding the patient's behavior, identifying their "suspicions" and asking whether the other party has noticed these or other behavioral changes in the individual.

  One should keep in mind that it is not uncommon for people to have a thought on "the tip of their tongue," which will generally be remembered later the same day. However, cognitively impaired individuals may not remember, even at a later time or date.

  Cognitively impaired individuals will often maintain good social skills—that is, they will be responsive to social exchanges such as "Hi, how are you?" and will reply, "Fine, and how are you?" They will often appear successful in "light" conversation, but, although their responses "sound" right, they may at times be inaccurate. For example, they may identify the wrong type of weather for the day or claim never to have been in the office before.

  Cognitively impaired individuals may complain of vague pain or discomfort but be unable to identify a specific location. Numerous tests or treatments may be recommended unnecessarily. When assessing an individual's pain, the practitioner should attempt to pinpoint the location, type of pain, duration, relief measures, and attempts to relieve it.

Having personal information available can be useful in maintaining a personal connection with the patient. This information should not be used as a true/false test but rather should be obtained as "new" information. For example, one should say to the patient, "Do you have any pets? If so, what kind and what are their names?"—asking for specifics that can be confirmed through the chart or by a caregiver. By contrast, "How is your dog Wrigley doing?" is a general question and allows for a nonspecific response, which is more difficult to assess for accuracy and confirm with the patient's record than is the previous query.

References

[1] Wilson RS, Beckett LA, Barnes LL, et al. Individual differences in rates of change in cognitive abilities of older persons. Psychol Aging 2002;17(2):179–93.

[2] Boeve B, McCormick J, Smith G, et al. Mild cognitive impairment in the oldest old. Neurology 2003;60(3):477–80.

[3] Moye J, Karel MJ, Azar AR, et al. Capacity to consent to treatment: empirical comparison of three instruments in older adults with and without dementia. Gerontologist 2004;44(2): 166–75.

[4] Kim SY, Karlawish JH, Caine ED. Current state of research on decision-making competence of cognitively impaired elderly persons. Am J Geriatr Psychiatry 2002;10(2):151–65.

[5] Bennett DA. Mild cognitive impairment. Clin Geriatr Med 2004;20(1):15–25.

[6] Crawford S, Channon S. Dissociation between performance on abstract tests of executive function and problem solving in real-life–type situations in normal aging. Aging Ment Health 2002;6(1):12–21.

[7] Hess TM, Rosenberg DC, Waters SJ. Motivation and representational processes in adulthood: the effects of social accountability and information relevance. Psychol Aging 2001;16(4):629–42.

[8] Rahhal TA, Colcombe SJ, Hasher L. Instructional manipulations and age differences in memory: now you see them, now you don't. Psychol Aging 2001;16(4):697–706.

[9] West R, Murphy KJ, Armilio ML, et al. Effects of time of day on age differences in working memory. J Gerontol B Psychol Sci Soc Sci 2002;57(1):3–10.

[10] Horn JL, Cattell RB. Age differences in fluid and crystallized intelligence. Acta Psychol (Amst) 1967;26(2):107–29.

[11] Katona CL. Psychotropics and drug interactions in the elderly patient. Int J Geriatr Psychiatry 2001;16(Suppl 1):S86–90.

[12] Mersulam M-M. Primary progressive aphasia—a language-based dementia. N Engl J Med 2003;349(16):1535–41.

[13] American Psychiatric Association. Diagnostic and Statistical Manual of Mental Disorders (DSM-IV). 4th edition. Washington, DC: American Psychiatric Association; 1994.

[14] Alva G, Potkin SG. Alzheimer disease and other dementias. Clin Geriatr Med 2003;19(4): 763–76.

[15] Mace NL, Rabins PV. The 36 hour day. New York: Warner Books; 2001.

[16] Freund B, Gravenstein S. Recognizing and evaluating potential dementia in office settings. Clin Geriatr Med 2004;20(1):1–14.

[17] Callahan CM, Hendrie HC, Tierney WM. Documentation and evaluation of cognitive impairment in elderly primary-care patients. Ann Intern Med 1995;122(6):422–9.

[18] Cummings JL. Fluctuations in cognitive function in dementia with Lewy bodies. Lancet Neurol 2004;3(5):266.

[19] Little JW, Falace DA. Dental management of the medically compromised patient. 4th edition. St. Louis (MO): Mosby-Year Book; 1993.

[20] Small GW, Rabins PV, Barry PP, et al. Diagnosis and treatment of Alzheimer disease and related disorders. Consensus statement of the American Association for Geriatric

Psychiatry, the Alzheimer's Association, and the American Geriatrics Society. JAMA 1997; 278(16):1363–71.

[21] Kral VA. Senescent forgetfulness: benign and malignant. Can Med Assoc J 1962;86:257–60.

[22] Flicker C, Ferris SH, Reisberg B. Mild cognitive impairment in the elderly: predictors of dementia. Neurology 1991;41(7):1006–9.

[23] Bennett DA, Wilson RS, Schneider JA, et al. Natural history of mild cognitive impairment in older persons. Neurology 2002;59(2):198–205.

[24] Jonker C, Hooyer C. The Amstel project: design and first findings. The course of mild cognitive impairment of the aged; a longitudinal 4-year study. Psychiatr J Univ Ott 1990; 15(4):207–11.

[25] Goldman WP, Morris JC. Evidence that age-associated memory impairment is not a normal variant of aging. Alzheimer Dis Assoc Disord 2001;15(2):72–9.

[26] Petersen RC, Smith GE, Waring SC, et al. Mild cognitive impairment: clinical characterization and outcome. Arch Neurol 1999;56(3):303–8.

[27] Ritchie K, Artero S, Touchon J. Classification criteria for mild cognitive impairment: a population-based validation study. Neurology 2001;56(1):37–42.

[28] Petersen RC, Doody R, Kurz A, et al. Current concepts in mild cognitive impairment. Arch Neurol 2001;58(12):1985–92.

[29] Unverzagt FW, Gao S, Baiyewu O, et al. Prevalence of cognitive impairment: data from the Indianapolis Study of Health and Aging. Neurology 2001;57(9):1655–62.

[30] Graham JE, Rockwood K, Beattie BL, et al. Prevalence and severity of cognitive impairment with and without dementia in an elderly population. Lancet 1997;349(9068):1793–6.

[31] Lyketsos CG, Lopez O, Jones B, et al. Prevalence of neuropsychiatric symptoms in dementia and mild cognitive impairment: results from the Cardiovascular Health Study. JAMA 2002; 288(12):1475–83.

[32] Griffith HR, Belue K, Sicola A, et al. Impaired financial abilities in mild cognitive impairment: a direct assessment approach. Neurology 2003;60(3):449–57.

[33] Tuokko H, Frerichs R, Graham J, et al. Five-year follow-up of cognitive impairment with no dementia. Arch Neurol 2003;60(4):577–82.

[34] Storandt M, Grant EA, Miller JP, et al. Rates of progression in mild cognitive impairment and early Alzheimer's disease. Neurology 2002;59(7):1034–41.

[35] Skoog I. Vascular aspects in Alzheimer's disease. J Neural Transm Suppl 2000;59:37–43.

[36] Aronson MK, Post DC, Guastadisegni P. Dementia, agitation, and care in the nursing home. J Am Geriatr Soc 1993;41(5):507–12.

[37] Evans DA, Hebert LE, Beckett LA, et al. Education and other measures of socioeconomic status and risk of incident Alzheimer disease in a defined population of older persons. Arch Neurol 1997;54(11):1399–405.

[38] Hebert LE, Scherr PA, Bienias JL, et al. Alzheimer disease in the US population: prevalence estimates using the 2000 census. Arch Neurol 2003;60(8):1119–22.

[39] Nussbaum RL, Ellis CE. Alzheimer's disease and Parkinson's disease. N Engl J Med 2003; 348(14):1356–64.

[40] Coyle JT. Use it or lose it—do effortful mental activities protect against dementia? N Engl J Med 2003;348(25):2489–90.

[41] Jost BC, Grossberg GT. The natural history of Alzheimer's disease: a brain bank study. J Am Geriatr Soc 1995;43(11):1248–55.

[42] Geldmacher DS, Whitehouse PJ. Evaluation of dementia. N Engl J Med 1996;335(5):330–6.

[43] Chatterjee A, Strauss ME, Smyth KA, et al. Personality changes in Alzheimer's disease. Arch Neurol 1992;49(5):486–91.

[44] Knopman DS, Berg JD, Thomas R, et al. Nursing home placement is related to dementia progression—experience from a clinical trial. Neurology 1999;52(4):714–8.

[45] Larson EB, Shadlen MF, Wang L, et al. Survival after initial diagnosis of Alzheimer disease. Ann Intern Med 2004;140(7):501–9.

[46] Campbell AJ, Busby WJ, Robertson MC, et al. Disease, impairment, disability and social handicap: a community based study of people aged 70 years and over. Disabil Rehabil 1994; 16(2):72–9.

[47] Rubin EH, Morris JC, Berg L. The progression of personality changes in senile dementia of the Alzheimer's type. J Am Geriatr Soc 1987;35(8):721–5.

[48] Geldmacher DS. Differential diagnosis of dementia syndromes. Clin Geriatr Med 2004; 20(1):27–43.

[49] Alzheimer's Association. 10 warning signs. Available at:http://www.alz.org/AboutAD/Warning.asp. Accessed October 2004.

[50] Tunzi M. Can the patient decide? Evaluating patient capacity in practice. Am Fam Physician 2001;64(2):299–306.

[51] Shuman SK, Bebeau MJ. Ethical and legal issues in special patient care. Dent Clin North Am 1994;38(3):553–75.

[52] Odom JG, Odom SS, Jolly DE. Informed consent and the geriatric dental patient. Spec Care Dentist 1992;12(5):202–6.

[53] Marsh FH. Informed consent and the elderly patient. Clin Geriatr Med 1986;2(3):501–10.

[54] Moye J, Karel MJ, Azar AR, et al. Capacity to consent to treatment: empirical comparison of three instruments in older adults with and without dementia. Gerontologist 2004;44(2): 166–75.

[55] Fellows LK. Competency and consent in dementia. J Am Geriatr Soc 1998;46(7):922–6.

[56] Feinberg LF, Whitlatch CJ. Are persons with cognitive impairment able to state consistent choices? Gerontologist 2001;41(3):374–82.

[57] Gerety MB, Chiodo LK, Kanten DN, et al. Medical treatment preferences of nursing home residents: relationship to function and concordance with surrogate decision-makers. J Am Geriatr Soc 1993;41(9):953–60.

[58] Marson DC, McInturff B, Hawkins L, et al. Consistency of physician judgments of capacity to consent in mild Alzheimer's disease. J Am Geriatr Soc 1997;45(4):453–7.

[59] Wetle T. Ethical issues in geriatric dentistry. Gerodontology 1987;6(2):73–8.

ELSEVIER
SAUNDERS

Dent Clin N Am 49 (2005) 411–427

THE DENTAL
CLINICS
OF NORTH AMERICA

Medication Use and Prescribing Considerations for Elderly Patients

Bradley R. Williams, PharmD, FASCP, CGP*,
Jiwon Kim, PharmD

*University of Southern California, School of Pharmacy, 1985 Zonal Avenue,
Los Angeles, CA 90089-9121, USA*

The US Census Bureau [1] estimates that approximately 34.7 million people of at least 65 years of age and 4.25 million people of at least 85 years of age live in the United States. These figures represent 12.6% and 1.6%, respectively, of the total population. By the year 2030, the percentages are anticipated to be 19.9% and 2.4%. This increased longevity, however, does not necessarily imply good health. Almost 30% of adults aged 65 years and older rate their health status as fair or poor. More than 30% of people aged 65 to 74 and almost 45% of people aged 75 and above experience some form of disability [2]. Among adults aged 65 years and older, the most common chronic conditions are arthritis, hypertension, respiratory illnesses, heart disease, diabetes, stroke, and cancer [3]. One common characteristic of these conditions is the importance of pharmacotherapy in their successful management.

Medication use by older adults

As would be expected from the prevalence of chronic disease in their population, older adults are heavy consumers of prescription medicines. According to estimates from the Medicare Current Beneficiary Survey, more than 70% of Medicare beneficiaries take at least one chronic medication, and nearly one third take at least three chronic medications. Almost 60% of community-dwelling elderly take at least three medicines [4]. Not unexpectedly, those who have more health problems take more drugs.

* Corresponding author.
E-mail address: bradwill@hsc.usc.edu (B.R. Williams).

Cardiovascular drugs are taken by more than 58% of older adults and represent the most frequently prescribed drug class. Analgesics are taken by 28.3%, central nervous system drugs (anticonvulsants, antiemetics, muscle relaxants) are taken by 13.1%, and psychotherapeutic agents and respiratory-tract drugs are each taken by 18% of the elderly population [4].

Age-associated physiologic changes affect the way older adults respond to drugs. Changes in gastric acidity and gastrointestinal motility can slow drug absorption and delay the onset of action of drugs, such as analgesics. Increased body fat and decreased body water and serum albumin levels modify the distribution patterns and alter the duration of action or pharmacologic activity of several agents, including sedatives and anesthetics. The reduced activity of many hepatic enzyme systems and decreased renal function may increase the risk for drug interactions and slow the elimination of medications [5].

Several other factors cause changes in drug response. Geriatric patients often are more susceptible than younger adults to central nervous system depressants. Reduced parasympathetic nervous system activity increases the likelihood that anticholinergic adverse effects will occur; the resulting dry mouth may adversely affect oral health [6]. The decline in the density of beta-adrenergic receptors can affect the vasodilatory response in the elderly. Reduced cardiac output and decreased total body water, combined with changes in baroreflexes, predispose older adults to hypotension and orthostatic effects of diuretics and antihypertensive agents; this should be considered when positioning elderly patients in a dental chair [7].

Polymedicine and medication-related problems

The risk that an adverse drug reaction or drug interaction will occur increases with the number of medications taken. The prevalence of medication use plus other factors predisposes older adults to medication-related problems (MRP). In addition to age-associated alterations in pharmacokinetics and pharmacodynamics, use of unnecessary or inappropriate medications and nonadherence to medication regimens contribute to the development of MRP. Age per se is probably not a factor for medication-related problems [8].

Polymedicine often is recognized as the use of more than a certain number of medications (eg, five or more). However, associating polymedicine only with the number of drugs taken can be misleading. An elderly patient who takes four drugs but who has only mild pain from osteoarthritis that is managed with acetaminophen may be exhibiting polymedicine. In contrast, a patient taking a total of eight medicines to treat diabetes mellitus, hypertension, hyperlipidemia, hypothyroidism, and rheumatoid arthritis may be living independently because of the use of multiple drugs. A more appropriate definition of polymedicine is the use of unnecessary medications, independent of the number of drugs taken. This definition directly links medication use to specific problems and allows for a better evaluation of a patient's drug regimen.

Several factors contribute to the development of polymedicine. The presence of multiple disease states often leads to the prescribing of several medications. The risk for adverse drug reactions or interactions increases with the number of medications, and the adverse reactions may then be treated with additional medications. A prescriber, unaware of drugs ordered by other clinicians, may prescribe a medication that duplicates or antagonizes the effect of a medicine the patient is already taking.

The use of medications that pose a high risk for adverse effects in older adults contributes to MRP. Potentially inappropriate medications are prescribed to more than one in five community-dwelling elderly people [9]. These are drugs that should be avoided in older adults because they either are ineffective, produce a high rate of adverse reactions, or are contraindicated in the presence of some diseases common among the elderly [10,11]. Examples of potentially inappropriate medications with relevance to dental practice are noted in Table 1. Prescription of potentially inappropriate medications to elderly patients has been estimated to occur during 4.45% to 7.8% of visits to physicians' offices in the United States [12,13]. Although there are no specific data on the likelihood of such practices occurring in dental offices, the figure may be quite similar.

Patients also contribute to MRP. Older adults are the most frequent consumers of nonprescription remedies and increasingly turn to alternative medicines to self-treat disease symptoms. Many older adults respond to advertising or rely on testimonials from friends or relatives to help them decide which product to purchase. In addition, direct-to-consumer advertising of prescription medications fuels the demand for products that are often new, expensive, and not well tested in the geriatric population. It is thus important that a medication history specifically include nonprescription and alternative medications to minimize the risks associated with self-treatment.

Polymedicine and nonadherence are frequently linked. Col et al [14] reported that 28% of admissions of older adults to a major medical center were due to medication-related problems. Adverse drug reactions were implicated in 60% of those admissions; nonadherence to medication regimens accounted for the remainder. Difficulty in recalling a medication regimen, multiple medications, multiple prescribers, female gender, moderate income, and the perception that medications were expensive were predictors for nonadherence. Fitten et al [15] identified diminished functional and cognitive capacities and increasing complexity of the medication regimen as factors predisposing elderly patients to nonadherence to medication regimens. The necessity of taking multiple daily doses also reduces adherence to a drug regimen [16].

Table 1
Problematic or potentially inappropriate medications for older adults

Medication	Potential problem
Analgesics	
Meperidine	CNS toxicity with oral dosage forms
NSAIDs	High risk of CNS effects (indomethacin); caution in patients with cardiovascular problems
Pentazocine	High risk of CNS adverse effects, ceiling analgesic effect
Propoxyphene (and combination)	Narcotic adverse effects; no better analgesia than acetaminophen
Psychotropic agents	
Benzodiazepines	Long-acting agents have prolonged effects; increased risk for falls and confusion
Phenotiazine antipsychotics	Sedation, dry mouth, dizziness, orthostatic hypotension, pseudoparkinsonism
Tricyclic antidepressants	Sedation, dry mouth, dizziness, orthostatic hypotension
Antihistamines	
Sedating agents	Chlorpheniramine, diphenhydramine, hydroxyzine, and promethazine have high anticholinergic properties.
Antispasmodics	
Bowel antispasmodics	Dry mouth, reduced gastrointestinal motility, changes in swallowing
Urinary bladder antispasmodics	Dry mouth, changes in swallowing

Abbreviations: CNS, central nervous system; NSAIDs, nonsteroidal anti-inflammatory drugs.

The most frequently prescribed medications in the elderly

The most frequently prescribed medications that may have an impact on dental treatment in older patients include cardiovascular drugs, anti-inflammatory agents, gastrointestinal agents, psychotropic agents, and endocrine agents [17]. Table 2 lists the most frequently prescribed medications in the elderly and the precautions dentists must take when delivering dental care to this patient population.

Cardiovascular drugs

Cardiovascular disease is the leading cause of death among people 65 years and older in the United States and one of the most common chronic disorders among elderly Americans [3]. Medications used to treat heart disease and other cardiovascular disorders include angiotensin-converting enzyme inhibitors (ACEIs), calcium channel blockers, beta-blockers, and diuretics and digoxin [18]. Warfarin is commonly used in geriatric patients with atrial fibrillation [19].

ACEIs are first-line agents for treating hypertension and heart failure in older patients [20,21]. ACEIs also are considered agents of choice in patients

Table 2
Most frequently prescribed medications and dental management considerations in the elderly

Drugs	Dental management considerations
Cardiovascular drugs	
Angiotensin-converting enzyme inhibitors	Angioedema, orthostatic hypotension, xerostomia
Calcium channel blockers	Orthostatic hypotension, xerostomia, gingival hyperplasia, drug interactions (erythromycin derivatives, bupivicaine, mepivicaine)
Beta blockers	Orthostatic hypotension, use of vasoconstrictors, xerostomia
Diuretics	Orthostatic hypotension, xerostomia
Digoxin	Orthostatic hypotension, drug interactions, xerostomia
Warfarin	Drug interactions, bleeding
Nonsteroidal anti-inflammatory drugs	
Nonspecific agents	Platelet inhibition, stomatitis
Cyclo-oxygenase-2 inhibitors	Platelet inhibition, stomatitis
Gastrointestinal agents	
Histamine-2 receptor antagonists	Xerostomia, regurgitation, altered taste, enamel erosion that can lead to pulpal disease
Proton pump inhibitors	Regurgitation, altered taste, pulpal disease, enamel erosion that can lead to pulpal disease
Psychotropic agents	
Benzodiazepines	Sedation, cognitive impairment, dry mouth
Selective serotonin reuptate inhibitors	Dizziness, dry mouth, taste changes

with diabetes. The most common side effects of ACEIs are dry cough, orthostatic hypotension, and dizziness. Angioedema is a rare but severe adverse effect associated with ACEIs [22].

Calcium channel blockers, such as amlodipine, nifedipine, diltiazem, and verapamil, also are used frequently for treatment of hypertension and chronic stable angina in older adults. Amlodipine and other long-acting dihydropyridine calcium channel blockers are considered the preferred treatment for the isolated systolic hypertension commonly seen in the elderly [23]. Common adverse effects of calcium channel blockers are flushing, peripheral edema, headache, and oral side effects, including dry mouth and gingival hyperplasia [24].

Diuretics are commonly prescribed to older patients for the control of hypertension and edema. Thiazides (eg, hydrochlorothiazide) are used primarily as first-line agents for hypertension, and the loop diuretics (eg, furosemide) are used to alleviate edema in congestive heart failure (CHF). Dehydration and electrolyte imbalances are common side effects of diuretics [18].

Digoxin is used in the management of atrial fibrillation and CHF but is associated with a narrow therapeutic index and can lead to digitalis toxicity, especially in elderly patients with compromised renal function. Symptoms of digoxin toxicity include nausea, confusion, and cardiac arrhythmias [18].

Warfarin is used to prevent stroke and other thromboembolic events in atrial fibrillation, which affects about 5% of the geriatric population. Several factors put elderly patients at increased risk for bleeding with warfarin therapy, including slower metabolic clearance of drugs, multiple chronic illnesses, and drug interactions [25]. Therefore, laboratory assessment of bleeding risk should be obtained before performing a dental procedure that will induce bleeding.

Antihypertensive agents, including diuretics, have been associated with xerostomia [26], which may induce oral pain, taste changes, and increased risk for oral infections such as gingivitis, oral candidiasis, and multiple dental caries. A thorough medication review and comprehensive clinical examination are essential to proper management of drug-induced xerostomia in elderly patients who are particularly at risk because of chronic multiple drug therapy. Along with palliative measures and aggressive caries prevention methods, effective management of xerostomia may require a physician consultation for appropriate drug dosing regimen or therapeutic drug substitution in older individuals. In patients taking ACEIs, complete extraoral and intraoral examination should be conducted to rule out the possibility of ACEI-induced angioedema, because several cases of late-onset ACEI-associated angioedema have been reported [27].

All antihypertensive agents can cause hypotension, and dentists should take care to avoid imbalance and dizziness that may precipitate falls in older patients. Dentists should allow patients to sit up slowly from a reclined position and remain seated for a few minutes before leaving the chair. In addition, a thorough medical and drug history may help to identify patients with uncontrolled hypertension and make it possible to avoid cerebrovascular accidents or myocardial infarction in these patients by taking blood pressure readings at each appointment. Local anesthetics with vasoconstrictors should be used with caution; repeated injections of epinephrine over a short period of time can increase blood pressure in these patients. Several antibiotics commonly prescribed by dentists, including erythromycin and tetracycline, can increase the anticoagulant effect of warfarin and potentially cause severe bleeding in patients on warfarin therapy [28]. Drug interactions with warfarin should be thoroughly assessed before one prescribes new drugs for dental treatment (Table 3).

Nonsteroidal anti-inflammatory drugs

Nonsteroidal anti-inflammatory drugs (NSAIDs) comprise a large group of compounds that provide analgesic, anti-inflammatory, and antipyretic effects. Older adults frequently are prescribed NSAIDs for osteoarthritis,

Table 3
Warfarin drug interactions with commonly prescribed medications in dental treatment

Interacting drug	Adverse effect
Erythromycin	↑ anticoagulation and ↑ risk for bleeding
Tetracycline	↑ anticoagulation and ↑ risk for bleeding
Metronidazole	↑ anticoagulation and ↑ risk for bleeding
Chloral hydrate	↑ anticoagulation and ↑ risk for bleeding
Barbiturates	↓ anticoagulation and ↑ risk for thromboembolism

the most common cause of disability in people over 75 years of age and the most common cause of immobility in older adults [29]. NSAIDs are effective in the management of pain and inflammation in geriatric patients who experience inadequate pain relief from acetaminophen. An estimated 50% of all NSAIDs produced are consumed by older adults seeking relief from osteoarthritis pain [30]. NSAIDs, however, cause several adverse effects, including gastrointestinal (GI) bleeding, impaired renal function, and platelet inhibition. The risk of serious GI complications with NSAIDs therapy increases with advanced age [31]. Advanced age is also a major risk factor for NSAID–induced renal toxicity, which often presents as sodium and water retention and an increased risk for hypertension [32]. When treating patients who are receiving chronic NSAID therapy, dentists should be aware of platelet inhibition effects of NSAIDs and take precautions for bleeding complications in surgical cases. When prescribing analgesics for pain and inflammation, one should conduct a thorough medication history to avoid therapeutic duplication of anti-inflammatory agents.

Gastrointestinal agents

Both histamine-2 receptor antagonists (H_2 blockers) and proton pump inhibitors (PPIs) are commonly prescribed in the elderly for management of heartburn associated with gastroesophageal reflux disease (GERD) and peptic ulcer disease (PUD). They also are frequently used by older patients on chronic NSAID therapy to prevent GI toxicities. All currently marketed H_2 blockers (cimetidine, famotidine, nizatidine, ranitidine) are available by prescription and as reduced-strength over-the-counter (OTC) products; many older adults self-treat GI symptoms with these agents. All H_2 blockers are eliminated renally, and side effects associated with the accumulation of H_2 blockers may be present in older adults who have renal impairment. Adverse effects associated with cimetidine accumulation include confusion, delirium, and hallucinations [33]. Cimetidine also interacts with several drugs that can lead to toxic effects. Plasma concentrations of theophylline, warfarin, and quinidine can increase as a result of metabolic inhibition by cimetidine, causing severe toxicity because of the narrow therapeutic range of these medications. Although the low doses approved for OTC labeling are unlikely to cause serious drug interactions, many older patients with compromised renal function may experience reduced clearance of cimetidine, and chronic drug therapy can lead to drug accumulation and the potential for adverse events.

Omeprazole is the only PPI available without a prescription. It is indicated for frequent heartburn and is approved for a 14-day course of therapy [34]. Esomeprazole, lansoprazole, pantoprazole, rabeprazole, and higher-dose omeprazole are available by prescription. PPIs are potent acid reducers with well-documented safety and efficacy for GERD and PUD [35]. In dental patients with chronic H_2 blockers or PPI therapy, dentists should examine the possibility of undercontrolled reflux disorders. These can present with taste changes and enamel erosion, which, if sufficiently severe, can lead to pulpal disease. In addition, a semisupine position on the dental chair should be considered for these patients to avert regurgitation.

Psychotropic agents

Sedatives and anxiolytics are widely used in older patients [4]. The use of benzodiazepines is estimated to be as high as 40% in adults greater than 65 years of age [36]. Benzodiazepines undergo hepatic degradation before being cleared from the body, and age-associated changes in pharmacokinetics and pharmacodynamics predispose geriatric patients to a greater risk for adverse effects, such as excessive sedation [37], cognitive impairment, and falls [38].

Depression is the most common mental illness among older adults, occurring in about 15% of the geriatric population [39]. Among several available and equally efficacious classes of antidepressants, selective serotonin reuptake inhibitors (SSRIs) are the best tolerated in the elderly and the most widely prescribed antidepressants in this population [40]. Currently marketed SSRIs are fluoxetine, citalopram, escitalopram, paroxetine, and sertraline. Common side effects associated with SSRIs are dizziness, insomnia, and gastric distress. Because these central nervous system (CNS) agents are well known to cause dizziness and may cause sedation, precautions should be taken when providing them to elderly dental patients to minimize the potential for falls and fractures.

Endocrine agents

Over 20% of older individuals are diagnosed with diabetes [41], and several drugs are used to control blood glucose in these patients. Sulfonylureas, such as glipizide and glyburide, are often used as first-line agents for newly diagnosed diabetes and are commonly prescribed in older diabetics. Hypoglycemia associated with sulfonylureas is a special concern for older individuals, especially in those with renal impairment, because these drugs have renal elimination pathways [42]. Other classes of widely used antidiabetic agents include metformin, thiazolidinediones (pioglitazone, rosiglitazone), and meglitinides (nateglinide, repaglinide). For patients taking any one of these antidiabetic agents, dentists should pay careful attention to any symptoms of hyperglycemia (visual blurring, thirst, urinary frequency) and hypoglycemia (tremor, headache, dizziness) before initiating dental treatment. Reminding patients to take their medications and eat before coming to the dental appointment is important in reducing the occurrence of these events.

Hypothyroidism is another common disorder in the older population and is effectively managed with levothyroxine. Adverse effects of levothyroxine include palpitations, tachycardia, and myocardial infarction in severe cases. Although dental treatment of older patients with hypothyroidism is safe, these patients may be at small risk for myxedema coma during complicated and stressful dental treatment: one of the important risk factors for myxedema coma is advanced age [43]. In addition, potentially dangerous arrhythmias can occur when vasoconstrictors are administered during dental procedures to patients taking thyroid hormone replacement [44].

Medications frequently prescribed by dentists

Several factors complicate the prescription of medications to older patients by dentists. Pharmacokinetic and pharmacodynamic alterations, as described earlier, are one important consideration. Dosage adjustments may be needed to avoid drug toxicity. Other factors dentists need to consider before prescribing medications to elderly patients are multiple disease states, currently prescribed drugs, the potential for therapeutic duplication, and potential adverse effects and drug interactions. All medications frequently prescribed by dentists, including antibiotics, analgesics, anti-inflammatory agents, and sedatives, should be used with caution in older patients to avoid adverse effects and unnecessary complications.

Antibiotics

Antibiotic classes commonly used in dentistry include penicillins, cephalosporins (eg, cephalexin), macrolides (eg, azithromycin), tetracyclines, metronidazole, and clindamycin. Most antibiotics can be safely used in older patients without dosage reduction; dose adjustment is usually not necessary when a single-dose antibiotic prophylaxis is required before a dental treatment. Penicillins, cephalosporins, and tetracyclines are eliminated through the kidney; hence a dose reduction may be required when a 1- or 2-week course of antibiotic therapy is anticipated in elderly patients with severe renal impairment [45]. Accumulation of penicillins and cephalosporins can cause seizures in severe cases, and tetracycline accumulation can cause liver toxicity. Clindamycin-associated GI problems such as diarrhea and colitis have a higher incidence in older patients [46]. Older patients should be counseled carefully on symptoms of colitis and instructed about proper management of GI complications when clindamycin is prescribed.

The elderly are especially susceptible to several drug interactions with antibiotics. Antibiotics such as erythromycin, tetracycline, and metronidazole, which can increase the anticoagulant effect of warfarin and cause bleeding, should be avoided when possible. Erythromycin and tetracycline should be avoided in patients taking digoxin, because these drugs can increase the digoxin serum level and lead to digitalis toxicity [47]. Other significant drug interactions of which the dentist should be aware include the potential for erythromycin to increase the serum concentrations of felodipine, possibly leading to hypotension and edema, and the potential of theophylline to cause toxic effects such as tachycardia, arrhythmias, and seizures [48]. A thorough medication history is required to assess the potential for adverse drug interactions with commonly prescribed antibiotics.

Analgesics

Acetaminophen (APAP) usually is the analgesic of choice in older adults, owing to its safety profile compared with other available agents [49]. The recommended maximum daily dose of APAP is 4 g in healthy adults. In older patients, however, APAP dosage generally should be limited to 2 to 3 g per day because of reduced hepatic function in older individuals and the drug's potential for hepatotoxic effects, especially in patients who drink more than two alcoholic beverages a day [32]. When recommending APAP or prescribing an opioid/APAP combination (eg, hydrocodone/APAP [Vicodin]) for pain in older patients, dentists should be aware that patients may be taking other OTC medications containing APAP for other indications (eg, cough and cold preparations) and should ensure that usage of APAP is limited to 3 g per day.

Tramadol is another nonopioid analgesic that can safely and effectively be used for mild to moderate orofacial pain. It often is used in patients in whom NSAIDs are contraindicated. Tramadol is generally considered to have equal efficacy to codeine and hydrocodone [50]. Although tramadol has a mechanism of action similar to that of opioids, common side effects associated with narcotics, such as somnolence and constipation, are reduced with tramadol. The usual daily maximum dose of tramadol is 400 mg, but in elderly patients daily maximum dose should be limited to 200 to 300 mg because of the risk of seizures with drug accumulation, especially in those with renal and hepatic impairment [50,51].

Opioids are used for the short-term management of moderate to severe orofacial pain. Codeine is a weak opioid and may not provide adequate analgesia. The use of propoxyphene should be avoided in the elderly because of its limited efficacy and the risk for neural and cardiac toxicity [10,50,52]. Meperidine also should be avoided in older adults because of the high potential for CNS side effects, especially in elderly patients with compromised renal function [10,11]. Anxiety, tremor, and seizures can occur with meperidine accumulation, even with short-term usage. Alternative agents, such as hydromorphone and morphine, which are without concerns for accumulation and toxicity in older patients, are preferred. Especially problematic side effects of opioids for older patients are constipation and sedation. Constipation is the most common side effect of narcotics and is especially difficult for older patients who may already be taking other constipation-causing medications (eg, calcium channel blocker). Sedative effects during the short-term use of narcotic analgesics can increase the risk of falls in older patients [50]. Dentists should be aware of possible opioid-associated constipation in older individuals and offer preventive measures when prescribing narcotic analgesics in this population.

Anti-inflammatory agents

For orofacial pain that involves inflammation, NSAIDs are recommended for initial management, because APAP and tramadol do not exert anti-inflammatory effects. The most common side effects associated with NSAIDs are GI adverse effects, including dyspepsia, erosions, and ulcerations. NSAIDs also cause fluid retention and peripheral edema owing to their potential for renal toxicity, although these are not as common as GI side effects. Dentists should use caution when prescribing these agents to elderly patients with CHF and hypertension. Newly available cyclooxygenase (COX-2) inhibitors, such as celecoxib, may be preferred in older patients because of the reduced risk for severe GI adverse events; however, the risk of renal toxicity is equivalent to that of conventional NSAIDs [32]. The need for NSAID use should be thoroughly assessed before prescribing these anti-inflammatory agents to older adults taking warfarin, because of the increased risk of bleeding. Patients taking NSAIDs and anticoagulant medications have a 12-fold greater risk of GI bleeding [53]. In these patients, APAP or tramadol is preferred [54]. A history of PUD or other erosive or ulcerative conditions also requires careful attention before NSAIDs are prescribed in older patients. GI prophylactic agents such as H_2 blockers or PPIs may be indicated in these patients if NSAID therapy is required; the lowest effective dose should be prescribed. Table 4 lists considerations for dentists when prescribing NSAIDs to older patients.

Sedatives

Sedatives commonly used in dental practice include benzodiazepines, barbiturates, and chloral hydrate. Diazepam has a long half-life in the elderly: 80 hours as compared with 20 hours in young adults [55]. This prolonged half-life is due to increased volume of distribution of the drug and

Table 4
Dental considerations when prescribing NSAIDs in the elderly

Clinical issue	Dental considerations
Adverse drug interactions	NSAIDs can decrease the effects of antihypertensive drugs.
	↑ Risk for bleeding with concurrent warfarin therapy
	Digoxin toxicity may occur with concurrent use.
Concurrent illnesses	Caution in patients with CHF
	Caution in patients with hypertension
	Caution in patients with PUD, GERD

causes a greater degree of CNS depression in older patients, increasing the risk for falls and fractures [56]. Other long-acting benzodiazepines that should be avoided in the elderly include flurazepam, chlordiazepoxide, and clonazepam [10]. Lorazepam, oxazepam, and temazepam are less lipid soluble and have a different metabolic fate from diazepam, leading to less accumulation; hence these are recommended for elderly patients. These benzodiazepines are also devoid of drug interactions that can increase the serum drug concentration and the risk for CNS and respiratory depression.

Barbiturates are not recommended in older patients, again because of their prolonged half-life in this population and their potential to cause more side effects than other sedatives [10]. Common side effects of barbiturates in elderly patients include drowsiness, lethargy, and severe CNS depression, which can lead to falls and fractures. Barbiturates are potent inducers of hepatic enzymes involved in metabolism of other drugs, and drug interactions with barbiturates can result in inappropriately low levels of other medications. Warfarin metabolism is significantly increased with concurrent barbiturate therapy, for example, an effect that can decrease the anticoagulant effect of warfarin and lead to increased risk for thromboembolic events.

Choral hydrate is considered a second- or third-line sedative agent in the elderly and should be used only for short periods. Chloral hydrate has a prolonged half-life and a potential for severe CNS depression, especially in patients with renal dysfunction; its use in moderate to severe renal impairment is not recommended [57]. Chloral hydrate is also not recommended for elderly patients with chronic obstructive pulmonary disease, severe cardiac conditions, or GI disease.

Local anesthetics

Common local anesthetics used in dentistry are amides—lidocaine, mepivacaine, prilocaine, articaine, and bupivacine. In general, local anesthetics can be safely used in geriatric patients when an appropriate dose is administered. Because of chronic health problems and age-related reduced hepatic function, blood concentrations of local anesthetics may be higher in elderly patients when the dose is calculated based on what is acceptable for the average adult. Although adverse drug reactions due to local anesthetics are unlikely after single-dose anesthetic therapy, dentists should proceed with caution, especially when administering combined local anesthetics (eg, lidocaine combined with bupivacine) to older patients [58]. Local anesthetic toxicity presenting as CNS excitation, convulsions, and respiratory depression has been reported with combination therapy exceeding recommended dosing guidelines [59]. Special care is required in older patients with hepatic disease, because the amides undergo hepatic metabolism. An increased half-life of lidocaine has been demonstrated in individuals aged 65 years or more compared with younger adults [60]. In addition, the inhibition of lidocaine metabolism by potent enzyme inhibitors, such as cimetidine, leads to a prolonged elevation of lidocaine blood concentration in geriatric patients, especially when high doses of lidocaine are used or repeated injections are required for prolonged dental procedures [58]. When using a local anesthetic combined with a vasoconstrictor in older patients, the physician should thoroughly review medical and drug histories to prevent possible adverse events. Epinephrine should be used with caution in hyperthyroid patients, because hypertensive crisis and cardiac arrhythmias are possible; likewise, care should be taken with diabetic patients because of their increased risk for hyperglycemia. Propranolol, a nonselective beta blocker, can lead to serious cardiovascular events when combined with a vasoconstrictor, and heart rate and blood pressure should be monitored in patients taking this drug [61]. No such adverse reactions have been associated with the more commonly used beta blockers metoprolol and atenolol.

Avoiding medication-related problems

Avoiding medication mishaps in elderly patients requires effort in several areas. The first steps are identifying and avoiding the use of medications that present a high risk for adverse reactions and identifying patients who are more likely to experience therapeutic misadventures. The Beers list [10] provides a good overview of medications that should be avoided in older adults. Many of the agents that compose the list are older agents that are not well tolerated, present a high risk for toxicity, and are equivalent or inferior to newer pharmacologic agents. They include long-acting benzodiazepines, meperidine, propoxyphene, and pentazocine. Caution is warranted when reviewing any list of potentially inappropriate medications; drugs not appearing on the list may, in fact, be highly dangerous when used in some individuals.

Certain populations of elderly patients are at greater risk than others for developing MRPs. Nursing facility residents take large numbers of medications, including psychotropic and cardiovascular medications that predispose them to cognitive impairment, falls, and other functional deficits

[62]. A similar pattern exists among older adults living in residential facilities for the elderly [63].

In any environment, patients with multiple diseases are at high risk for MRPs, because of the frequent use of many medications and the likelihood that several practitioners are prescribing them without full knowledge of the patient's concurrent medication use. The risk for medication mishaps can be minimized by incorporating some simple strategies into the office visit routine for geriatric patients:

- Obtain a medication history for older patients. This should include prescription and nonprescription drugs, herbal medications, and dietary supplements. The list should be updated at every visit or at least annually.
- Review the history for medications that may potentially duplicate or antagonize medications prescribed in the dental office. Analgesic agents the patient is taking may be sufficient to treat pain that occurs after a procedure. NSAIDs should be avoided in patients taking warfarin or other agents that affect coagulation. A sedative prescribed by the primary physician may substitute for a preprocedural anxiolytic or sedative.
- Review the medication list for medications that have a negative effect on oral health. Many different medications have anticholinergic activity that may cause dry mouth or affect swallowing. A combination of several of these can lead to significant adverse effects.
- Use the primary care physician to coordinate care. Because the primary physician will probably see the patient most frequently, he or she should be notified if any significant addition is made to a medication regimen.
- Encourage the use of a single pharmacy. Pharmacists maintain patient medication profiles, so the use of a single pharmacy ensures that one location will have a record of all medications being taken by an older patient. When the pharmacist identifies a potential adverse reaction or drug interaction, he or she can contact the appropriate prescribers. The pharmacist can also evaluate and recommend nonprescription products for oral hygiene or therapy or refer the patient back to the dentist, when appropriate.

The care of many older adults is medically complex. Collaboration and communication between the dentist, patient, and other health care providers are essential to maximizing drug therapy outcomes and avoiding medication misadventures.

References

[1] Day JC. Population projects of the United States by age, sex, race, and Hispanic origin: 1995 to 2000. Washington, DC: U.S. Bureau of the Census, Current Population Reports, P25-1130, U.S. Government Printing Office; 1996.

[2] Blackwell DL, Tonthat L. Summary health statistics for the US population: National Health Interview Survey, 1999. National Center for Health Statistics. Vital Health Stat 10 2003;211:12–7.

[3] Adams PF, Hendershot GE, Marano MA. Current estimates from the National Health Interview Survey. 1996. National Center for Health Statistics. Vital Health Stat 10 1999; 200:81–2.

[4] Moxey ED, O'Connor JP, Novielli KD, et al. Prescription drug use in the elderly: a descriptive analysis. Health Care Financ Rev 2003;24(2):127–41.

[5] Yuen GJ. Altered pharmacokinetics in the elderly. Clin Geriatr Med 1990;6(2):257–68.

[6] Vargas CM, Kramarow EA, Yellowitz JA. The oral health of older Americans. Aging Trends, No. 3. Hyattsville (MD): National Center for Health Statistics; 2001.

[7] Feely J, Coakley D. Altered pharmacodynamics in the elderly. Clin Geriatr Med 1990;6(2): 269–84.

[8] Gurwitz JH, Avorn J. The ambiguous relation between aging and adverse drug reactions. Ann Intern Med 1991;114(11):956–66.

[9] Zhan C, Sangl J, Bierman AS, et al. Potentially inappropriate medication use in the community-dwelling elderly. JAMA 2001;286(22):2823–9.

[10] Beers MH. Explicit criteria for determining potentially inappropriate medication use by the elderly. Arch Intern Med 1997;157(14):1531–6.

[11] Fick DM, Cooper JW, Wade WE, et al. Updating the Beers criteria for potentially inappropriate medication use in older adults. Arch Intern Med 2003;163(22):2716–24.

[12] Aparasu RR, Sitzman SJ. Inappropriate prescribing for elderly outpatients. Am J Health Syst Pharm 1999;56(5):433–9.

[13] Goulding MR. Inappropriate medication prescribing for elderly ambulatory care patients. Arch Intern Med 2004;164(3):305–12.

[14] Col N, Fanale JE, Kronholm P. The role of medication noncompliance and adverse drug reactions in hospitalization of the elderly. Arch Intern Med 1990;150(4):841–5.

[15] Fitten LJ, Coleman L, Siembieda DW, et al. Assessment of capacity to comply with medication regimens in older adults. J Amer Geriatr Soc 1995;43(4):361–7.

[16] Eisen SA, Miller DK, Woodward RS, et al. The effect of prescribed daily dose frequency on patient medication compliance. Arch Intern Med 1990;150(9):1881–4.

[17] Paunovich ED, Sadowsky JM, Carter P. The most frequently prescribed medications in the elderly and their impact on dental treatment. Dent Clin North Am 1997;41(4): 699–726.

[18] Williams BR, Kim J. Cardiovascular drug therapy in the elderly: theoretical and practical considerations. Drugs Aging 2003;20(6):445–63.

[19] Feinberg WM, Blackshear JL, Laupacis A, et al. Prevalence, age distribution, and gender of patients with atrial fibrillation: analysis and implications. Arch Intern Med 1995;155(5): 469–73.

[20] Israili ZH, Hall WD. ACE inhibitors: differential use in elderly patients with hypertension. Drugs Aging 1995;7(5):355–71.

[21] Anonymous. Heart failure: evaluation and treatment of patients with left ventricular systolic dysfunction. Agency for Health Care Policy and Research (AHCPR). J Am Geriatr Soc 1998;46(4):525–9.

[22] Candelria LN, Hutula CS. Angioedema associated with angiotensin-converting enzyme inhibitors. J Oral Maxillofac Surg 1991;49(11):1237–9.

[23] Chobanian AV, Bakris GL, Black HR, et al. Joint National Committee on Prevention, Detection, Evaluation, and Treatment of High Blood Pressure. National Heart, Lung, and Blood Institute. National High Blood Pressure Education Program Coordinating Committee. Seventh report of the Joint National Committee on Prevention, Detection, Evaluation, and Treatment of High Blood Pressure. Hypertens 2003;42(6):1206–52.

[24] Hassell TM, Hefti AF. Drug induced gingival overgrowth: old problem, new problem. Crit Rev Oral Biol Oral Med 1991;2(1):103–37.

[25] Gurwitz JH, Avorn J, Ross-Degnan D, et al. Aging and the anticoagulant response. Ann Intern Med 1992;116(11):901–4.

[26] Madinier I, Jehl-Pietri C, Monteil RA. Drug-induced xerostomia. Ann Med Interne (Paris) 1997;148(5):398–405.

[27] Guo X, Dick L. Late onset angiotensin-converting enzyme induced angioedema: case report and review of the literature. J Okla State Med Assoc 1999;92(2):71–3.

[28] Hersh EV. Adverse drug interactions in dental practice: interactions involving antibiotics. Part II of a series. J Am Dent Assoc 1999;130(2):236–51.

[29] Felson DT. An update on the pathogenesis and epidemiology of osteoarthritis. Radiol Clin North Am 2004;42(1):1–9.

[30] Fries JF, Miller SR, Spitz PW, et al. Toward an epidemiology of gastropathy associated with nonsteroidal anti-inflammatory drug use. Gastroenterology 1989;96(2 Pt 2 Suppl):647–55.

[31] Hernandez-Diaz S, Rodriguez LA. Association between nonsteroidal anti-inflammatory drugs and upper gastrointestinal tract bleeding/perforation: an overview of epidemiologic studies published in the 1990s. Arch Intern Med 2000;160(14):2093–9.

[32] Gloth FM. Pain management in older adults: prevention and treatment. J Am Geriatr Soc 2001;49(2):188–99.

[33] Feldman M, Burton ME. Histamine2–receptor antagonists. Standard therapy for acid-peptic diseases. N Engl J Med 1990;323(25):1749–55.

[34] Anonymous. Over-the-counter omeprazole (Prilosec OTC). Med Lett Drugs Ther 2003; 45(1162):61–2.

[35] Vergara M, Vallve M, Gisbert JP, et al. Meta-analysis: comparative efficacy of different proton-pump inhibitors in triple therapy for Helicobacter pylori eradication. Aliment Pharmacol Ther 2003;18(6):647–54.

[36] Reynolds CF III, Kupfer DJ, Hoch CC, et al. Sleeping pills for the elderly: are they ever justified? J Clin Psychiatry 1985;46(2 Pt 2):9–12.

[37] Wang PS, Bohn RL, Glynn RJ, et al. Hazardous benzodiazepine regimens in the elderly: effects of half-life, dosage, and duration of risk of hip fracture. Am J Psychiatry 2001;158(6): 892–8.

[38] Greenblatt DJ, Harmatz JS, Shader RI. Clinical pharmacokinetics of anxiolytics and hypnotics in the elderly (Part 1). Clin Pharmacokinet 1991;21(3):165–77.

[39] Jeste DV, Alexopoulos GS, Bartels SJ, et al. Consensus statement on the upcoming crisis in geriatric mental health: research agenda for the next 2 decades. Arch Gen Psychiatry 1999; 56(9):848–53.

[40] Montgomery SA. Late-life depression: rationalizing pharmacological treatment options. Gerontology 2002;48(6):392–400.

[41] Harris MI, Hadden WC, Knowler WC, et al. Prevalence of diabetes and impaired glucose tolerance and plasma glucose levels in US population aged 20–74 yr. Diabetes 1987;36(4): 523–34.

[42] Brodows RG. Benefits and risks with glyburide and glipizide in elderly NIDDM patients. Diabetes Care 1992;15(1):75–80.

[43] Olsen CG. Myxedema coma in the elderly. J Am Board Fam Pract 1995;8(5):376–83.

[44] Naftalin LW, Yagiela JA. Vasoconstrictors: indications and precautions. Dent Clin North Am 2002;46(4):733–46.

[45] Gleckman RA, Czachor JS. Reviewing the safe use of antibiotics in the elderly. Geriatrics 1989;44(7):33–6.

[46] Neu HC, Prince A, Neu CO, et al. Incidence of diarrhea and colitis associated with clindamycin therapy. J Infect Dis 1977;135(Suppl):S120–5.

[47] Maxwell DL, Gilmour-White SK, Hall MR. Digoxin toxicity due to interaction of digoxin with erythromycin. BMJ 1989;298(6673):572.

[48] Gurevitz SL. Erythromycin: drug interactions. J Dent Hyg 1997;71(4):159–61.

[49] Tomaselli CE. Pharmacotherapy in the geriatric population. Spec Care Dentist 1992;12(3): 107–11.

[50] AGS Panel on Persistent Pain in Older Adults. Management of persistent pain in older adults. J Am Geriatr Soc 2002;50(Suppl):S205–24.

[51] Nightingale SL. From the Food and Drug Administration. JAMA 1996;275(16):1224.

[52] Davis MP, Srivastava M. Demographics, assessment and management of pain in the elderly. Drugs Aging 2003;20(1):23–57.

[53] Piper JM, Ray WA, Daugherty JR, et al. Corticosteroid use and peptic ulcer disease: role of nonsteroidal anti-inflammatory drugs. Ann Intern Med 1991;114(9):735–40.

[54] Phero JC, Becker D. Rational use of analgesic combinations. Dent Clin North Am 2002; 46(4):691–705.

[55] Greenblatt D, Allen M, Harmatz V. Diazepam disposition determinants. Clin Pharmacol Ther 1980;27(3):301–12.

[56] Closser MH. Benzodiazepines and the elderly: a review of potential problems. J Subst Abuse Treat 1991;8(1–2):35–41.

[57] Bennett WM, Aronoff GR, Golper TA, et al. Drug prescribing in renal failure. Philadelphia: American College of Physicians; 1987.

[58] Moore PA. Adverse drug interactions in dental practice: interactions associated with local anesthetics, sedatives, and anxiolytics. Part IV of a series. J Am Dent Assoc 1999;130(4): 541–54.

[59] Moore PA. Preventing local anesthesia toxicity. J Am Dent Assoc 1992;123(9):60–4.

[60] Nation RL, Triggs EJ, Selig M. Lignocaine kinetics in cardiac patients and aged subjects. Br J Clin Pharmacol 1977;4(4):439–48.

[61] Yagiela JA. Adverse drug reactions in dental practice: interactions associated with vasoconstrictors. Part V of a series. J Am Dent Assoc 1999;130(5):701–9.

[62] Williams BR, Thompson JF, Brummel-Smith KV. Improving medication use in the nursing home. In: Rubenstein LZ, Wieland D, editors. Improving care in the nursing home: comprehensive reviews of clinical research. Newbury Park (CA): Sage Publications; 1993. p. 33–64.

[63] Williams BR, Nichol MB, Lowe B, et al. Medication use in residential care facilities for the elderly. Ann Pharmacother 1999;33(2):149–55.

ELSEVIER
SAUNDERS

THE DENTAL
CLINICS
OF NORTH AMERICA

Dent Clin N Am 49 (2005) 429–443

Caring for Elderly Long-Term Care Patients: Oral Health–Related Concerns and Issues

Michael I. MacEntee, LDS(I),
Dip Prosth, FRCD(C), PhD

*Faculty of Dentistry, University of British Columbia, 2199 Wesbrook Mall,
Vancouver, BC, Canada V6T 1Z3*

The population everywhere is aging at a remarkable rate, and the expected increase in the number of very old people (>80 years) is stunning in most countries, whether rich or poor. For instance, 16% of Europeans and 13% of North Americans were over 65 years of age in 2000, whereas 3% of the population in both regions was older than 80 years [1]. The projected increase in actual numbers of very old people—currently more than 9 million in the United States—draws attention to the need for more information about them. This aging population has been expanding for several decades and will continue to do so for the foreseeable future. The legacy of a low fertility rate during the 1914 to 1918 war restrained the growth rate of the "oldest-old" (ie >80 years) to about 1% between 1996 and 1997, after which it rose to 3.5% between 1997 and 2000 (versus 2% for the >65 group) when those born after 1918 reached 80. This growth is currently expected to remain above 3% for the next 10 to 15 years. Today, about one in four elderly Americans (>65 years) and one in five elderly Japanese are more than 80 years of age, a ratio that should remain constant for a quarter century. Other countries have smaller ratios of people aged older than 80 to people aged older than 65, but they too expect a noticeable increase over the next few years.

Life expectancy at birth for a man or woman in North America was about 60 years during the early part of the last century, whereas today it is over 75 years in most industrialized countries, with Japan topping the list at 76 years for men and 84 years for women [1]. Even in old age, life expectancies continue to improve because of a slower progression of chronic

E-mail address: macentee@interchange.ubc.ca

0011-8532/05/$ - see front matter © 2005 Elsevier Inc. All rights reserved.
doi:10.1016/j.cden.2004.10.008

diseases [2]. On retiring at age 65, healthy women now expect at least 20 years and healthy men 16 years; they can all look toward another 5 or 6 years on their 85th birthdays [3].

These facts translate into a substantial increase in the number of very old people who will need special care and attention to maintain a reasonable quality of life in the face of disability and growing frailty. The net result is that demands for health and social services will increase substantially over the next quarter century [4].

Frailty and long-term care recipients

The typical resident of a long-term care (LTC) facility uses seven or more prescribed medications daily for hypertension, heart disease, and a variety of other ailments [5]. However, it is the increasing lapses of memory, restricted mobility, hearing loss, poor eyesight, and insomnia that pose the greatest challenge to an older person's independence. Ultimately, the need for special nursing follows the impact of chronic disability and frailty, so that about one third of the population older than 80 and half of those older than 90 move to the protective environment of an LTC facility [6,7]. The apparent decline over the past few decades in the number of people entering the traditional nursing home or LTC facility—currently about 6% of 65 year olds—can be accounted for in part by a proliferation of other health care settings for older people (eg, "assisted living facilities," "continuing care facilities") that provide some form of residential care [8]. Government policies in many jurisdictions prescribe the expected quality of care in facilities to promote health, safety, and overall quality of life [9]. But it is not uncommon to find that regulations are intentionally vague in ethical deference to personal choice and the rights of the individual. Several jurisdictions in Canada [10,11] and the United States [12] regulate that the mouths of all new residents be examined soon after admission to an LTC facility, but they do not specify who should perform the examination, nor do they insist on follow-up treatment [13,14]. Only one in five (19%) of the nursing home residents in the United States received dental services in 1997, although the government aims to improve the ratio to one in four by 2010 [15].

Oral health status of frail elders

Numerous epidemiologic investigations attest to the low priority given to oral health in many LTC facilities and to the consequences of this neglect [16–21]. Few indications exist that the problem has been addressed effectively over the last quarter century, despite increasing awareness among dental professionals, nursing staff, and health care administrators [22–24]. Worse still, evidence suggests that concern for oral health, never strong in this setting [25], has actually deteriorated, even among dentists and dental hygienists [26–28]. A recent survey of all (>2000) dentists in British

Columbia, for example, found that only 43 respondents had any interest in attending to the residents of LTC facilities, and a little more than half (n = 26) of them were providing this service (Association of Dental Surgeons of British Columbia, personal communication, 2004). By contrast, the administrators of nearly half (43%) of the 294 facilities in the province asked for help in improving the oral health of their residents. The responses of the dentists were not much different from those obtained about 30 years ago [25,26]. Dentists appear to believe that financial constraints, the apathy of residents and staff, uncooperative administrators, and inadequate clinical equipment are partially to blame, although they acknowledge that their own limited educational experience and clinical involvement in LTC do little to rectify the situation [29]. Similarly, a survey of physicians in the American Medical Association revealed that only one third of the respondents spent any measurable time caring for nursing home residents [30]. Clearly, the lack of interest in LTC is not unique to dentistry.

Preventive and treatment strategies

Emergency and diagnostic services

On a more optimistic note, the author can report that some dental professionals and administrators of LTC facilities are cooperating to tackle the diagnostic, emergency, and ongoing oral treatment needs of frail elders. As yet, there is no consensus on an appropriate strategy of care [31–33]. Administrators almost unanimously agree that residents must have access to dental emergency care when it is necessary to manage pain and infection. Many of them acknowledge their legal responsibility to provide an oral diagnostic service from a dental professional before pathos, disease, or dysfunction causes irreparable damage [23]. Consequently, many facilities have arrangements with a dentist or dental hygienist to provide emergency care and the occasional diagnostic service, although they are much less prepared to provide the ongoing care received by most independent adults in Western society.

Caries

Tooth loss in old age is primarily a consequence of caries [34], either directly through active demineralization of coronal and root surfaces (ie, active caries) or indirectly and more typically from endodontic pathoses or tooth fracture. The risk for caries continues into old age, particularly when medications disturb saliva and the frequency of sugar consumption is high. Frail elders are at particular risk for caries because of the constant availability of sugary snacks—such as muffins—because of their impaired ability to clear residual food from the mouth during meals, and because of saliva that is limited both in quantity and buffering capacity [35,36]. Cariogenic food may remain in contact with teeth for most of the day and night, causing the teeth to demineralize unless fluoride has increased their resistance. It is much more difficult to change the dietary habits of an LTC facility, despite the evidence that prolonged exposure to sugars and other refined carbohydrates damages teeth.

The damage caused by caries in old age can be devastating, although more rampant attacks are confined, as in childhood, to a few highly susceptible individuals. In a longitudinal study over 2 years, frail elders with very poor oral hygiene and abundant dental plaque had on average 14 teeth—6 carious and 6 restored—at the beginning of the study, yet only one subject in the first year and two subjects in the second year developed more than two new or recurrent carious lesions [37]. One subject had seven new lesions in the first year and 13 in the second year; another developed 19 new lesions in the first year alone. Overall, the average net incidence per person was 0.9 carious surfaces during year 1 and 3.4 surfaces during year 2. If the two individuals with most of the new carious surfaces were excluded from the analysis, the net incidence dropped to 1.8 lesions per person over the 2 years. In fact, the general health of the subjects deteriorated more rapidly than their teeth; the caries caused little discomfort or tooth loss, and the new or recurrent caries developed independently of fluoride use (no fluoride was present in the local water supply), tooth extractions, or tooth restorations. Small studies such as this one throw only a little light on the dynamic nature of the mouth, and much larger studies are required to identify the specific factors influencing oral health in the midst of rapidly progressing frailty. Other authors, by contrast, have reported that elderly people who lived a long time in fluoridated communities had less caries than those from nonfluoridated areas [38]. Reports on caries tend to overlook the dynamic nature of the mouth: lesions can recalcify or reverse as others form, and rampant caries is usually restricted to a few highly susceptible individuals.

An ozone-generating device for eliminating *Streptococcus mutans* and *Streptococcus sobrinus* from root lesions in old teeth shows promise [39]. A strong concentration (10%) of chlorhexidine in a varnish applied frequently to the teeth (once per week for 4 weeks and once again at 6 months) did inhibit the incidence of root caries in functionally independent adults with salivary disorders [40]. For the foreseeable future, however, mouth rinses or sponges containing fluoride probably offer the most practical strategy for controlling caries in functionally dependent elders [41], although more research is needed to confirm the effectiveness of the products [42]. A randomized clinical trial comparing daily mouth rinses with 0.2% neutral sodium fluoride, 0.12% chlorhexidine, or a placebo solution among 116 residents of several LTC facilities over 2 years resulted in a mean increase of only 0.7 carious surfaces in the fluoride group, which was significantly less than the three carious surfaces found in both of the other groups [43]. Neutral fluoride is preferable to acidulated or stannous products for older adults, because it does not damage or stain ceramic or acrylic prostheses [44], and toxicity is unlikely even when the full content of a mouth rinse bottle is swallowed [45]. As cognitive awareness declines, some people will have difficulty rinsing the mouth without swallowing the rinse. In this situation, the fluoridated rinse can be applied sparingly to the teeth with a sponge.

Restorative treatment

No consensus exists on how best to render dental restorative treatment to people who cannot easily leave home. Dentists prefer to have nursing home residents transported to a fully equipped dental clinic, whereas the residents, their families, and the facility's staff usually request dental treatment within the home. Moving a frail resident to attend a dentist can be stressful for everyone involved and is probably a major reason why many restorative treatment suggestions are readily rejected. Moreover, little or no evidence supports the overall effectiveness of dental services to this population, regardless of where they are rendered [13,46].

Prosthodontics

Although loss of all natural teeth is not a natural consequence of aging, about one third of persons over 65 and most of those over 75 have lost all of their natural teeth [47,48]. A remarkable decline in tooth loss has occurred over the last few decades [49], although complete or partial tooth loss and the need to replace some teeth remain facts of life for almost all older adults [50,51]. Adults with fewer than 20 teeth experience a significant decline in oral comfort and nutritional intake [52]. Therefore, a reasonable objective of prosthodontic treatment is to restore or replace the dentition so that anterior teeth have an acceptable appearance and posterior teeth provide bilateral contacts for chewing comfortably [53–56].

Identification of removable dentures is necessary in nursing homes to prevent their loss. It is a simple and, in some jurisdictions, a required process to place a visible identification mark on or beneath the surface of a denture base [57]. It is best to place the identification within the denture base under clear acrylic resin when the denture is made, but a mark with an indelible pen on the surface of the base, although less durable, can be effective.

Oral implants

Age has no detrimental effect on the success of endosseous oral implants [58], and some experts advocate the two-implant overdenture as the primary standard of care for all edentulous people [59]. Therefore, the number of people with implant-supported dentures who are frail and dependent on others for daily care is growing. As yet, the number is small and little information is available about problems associated with the implants or the dentures. Nonetheless, we do know that the prosthodontic maintenance associated with implants can be complicated, time consuming, and expensive

[60,61], and it is likely that in the near future this problem will add to the difficulties of managing oral health in LTC.

Gingivitis and periodontal disease

A sense is emerging that the usual measures of dental plaque used to predict gingivitis among younger adults may be inappropriate for frail elders. Frail elders appear less concerned in general than their less disabled contemporaries about food debris, bacterial plaque, and gingivitis around their teeth, probably because of reduced proprioceptive awareness in or around the mouth [62]. This diminished awareness may be significant to general health if, in fact, bacterial plaque and oral debris are linked to aspiration pneumonia, as some studies suggest [63,64]. The status of this claim awaits the outcome of further clinical investigations, but the proposed micropathologic connection between oral and pulmonary bacteria is plausible.

Severe periodontitis is uncommon in older people with natural teeth, despite poor oral hygiene and the pervasiveness of gingivitis [65]. Nearly everyone loses some periodontal attachment over time; however, it is very unusual for the loss to occur rapidly in old age. Consequently, the need for treatment strategies to control periodontal disease, in contrast to gingival inflammation, is low among elderly residents of LTC facilities.

Oral hygiene

Concerns about general oral hygiene cause significant distress to everyone involved in LTC. Administrators, nurses, and care aides are all aware of the need to help clean the teeth of the residents in their care, but they acknowledge that the mouth is neglected because of the many other demands on their time [23]. Dentists and dental hygienists also feel frustrated by the challenge of providing oral hygiene in this environment. In general, support for oral health care varies from facility to facility. Residents cannot get toothbrushes or toothpaste without great difficulty in some facilities, whereas administrators in others have appointed "oral care specialists" from among their fulltime staff to champion dental matters [24]. The mix of care staff from various sociocultural and educational backgrounds, together with the various and inconsistent expectations of residents, compounds the problem of oral hygiene in LTC. Furthermore, there is a strong sense in most societies today that the autonomy of dependent persons must be respected as much as possible, even when they refuse help with personal hygiene. Hence the problem of oral hygiene is acknowledged widely, even if solutions are not yet readily available.

Dentures are not always cleaned effectively to remove the bacteria and fungi associated with stomatitis. With increasing frailty, the risk of aspiration pneumonia is probably substantially increased when accumulations of oral bacteria and fungi are high [63,64]. Denture wearers usually are advised to soak their dentures in a cleansing solution, such as alkaline peroxides or sodium hypochlorite. The peroxide products are widely available from pharmacies and reasonably effective. Alternatively, household bleach (sodium hypochlorite) in a *dilute* solution of one part 5% sodium hypochlorite to three parts water can be used for dentures made solely of acrylic resin.[1] Generally, soaking a denture for 30 minutes a day in an effervescent peroxide solution or in a dilute bleach will suffice if the denture is also brushed thoroughly with soap and water.

It is not always possible for disabled people to brush a denture effectively; hence, the effectiveness of chemical solutions and other methods of removing plaque and disinfecting acrylic resin are being investigated. For example, a short-term clinical study in nursing homes of three effervescent denture cleansers found that they all had a similar advantage over water in reducing stains, calculus, bacteria, and fungi [66]. Traditionally, denture wearers have been advised to soak their dentures in water when the dentures were not in use. However, evidence suggests that the bacterial and fungal contamination of dentures is much reduced when the dentures are dry when not in use [67]. Apparently, a wet environment promotes bacterial and fungal growth, whereas concerns about the distortion of acrylic resin when allowed to dry are of no clinical concern.

Another study demonstrated the effectiveness of irradiating dentures in a microwave oven for one minute at 850 watts [68]. This method might be an effective and efficient way of inoculating dentures for people who are at particular risk for pneumonia, but the investigators warned against using microwaves on dentures that have been repaired or relined or on ceramic teeth with metallic pins. In the United States, the Food and Drug Administration is required to approve all sterilization equipment [69], and microwave units are currently not subject to this approval; hence this may not be a viable method of sterilizing acrylic dentures in the United States.

The hygiene needed to maintain an implant denture is not radically different from the hygiene needed for gingival health. The bars attached to implants beneath removable dentures and the pontics of fixed prostheses require good manual dexterity and knowledge of structural design for effective cleaning. Fortunately, accumulations of plaque around implants do not influence the success or failure of the implants in bone [70]. They do, however, cause halitosis and a mucositis that is locally and psychologically irritating. Poor oral hygiene and halitosis are a major concern of older people who are relatively healthy, because these conditions are associated with poor general health and unacceptable social behavior [71].

---

[1] Bleach in full concentration will "whiten" acrylic resin and corrode the base metal alloys in removable partial denture.

Educational programs to prevent disease

The Brief Oral Health Status Examination [72], the Index of Activities of Daily Oral Hygiene [73], and the Index of Clinical Oral Disorder in Elders [74] have been developed to assess oral health in an LTC setting. They all need further development and testing to confirm their value as predictors of oral health and to enhance their use by nurses, care aides, and other nondental personnel. Care aides and nurse in the United States are required to access oral health as part of the Minimum Data Set collected on all new admissions to LTC facilities [12], but the results are inconsistent because of different educational backgrounds and the lack of a standardized approach to the examinations [75,76].

Innovative attempts have been made to educate nurses and care aides about recognizing oral diseases and about oral hygiene for residents who are profoundly disabled, but here too the results are inconclusive [77–79]. Some interventions produced clinical benefit for the residents [80], some enhanced the knowledge of the nursing staff [81,82], and others had scarcely any measurable benefits [83]. Moreover, when a course of instruction did raise enthusiasm for oral care among nursing staff, it was short-lived [79,84]. Unfortunately, all the studies on educational interventions have been limited by uncertainty about the clinical measures available for assessing appropriate levels of oral hygiene and comfort and by the difficulties of research in the complicated environment of an LTC facility.

Propensity for treatment

Partial tooth replacement based on the concept of a "minimal threshold" or a "shortened dental arch" [85] raises issues related to the propensity for treatment in old age. Essentially, the phrase "propensity for treatment" addresses the need to consider disabled people in the context of their physical and cognitive abilities, their overall desire for treatment, and their ability to benefit from it. It assigns particular relevance to quality of life, given the likelihood that dental treatment will benefit self-image and social interaction more than physical function [86,87]. In general, elders seek treatment for problems that they believe are serious and likely to be treated successfully [62]. However, the significance attached to a specific problem changes as frailty increases and the propensity for treatment declines. This pattern holds particularly true in the LTC facility, with its many conflicting priorities and cultural pressures [23,24]. Analysis of information collected from the residents of facilities in Vancouver found that one in three had the propensity for comprehensive dental treatment and was probably capable of benefiting from it; one in ten was so disabled that he or she was not interested in dental treatment under most circumstances and was unlikely to benefit from it, and the rest might have benefited from a conservative or minimally invasive approach to treatment [50]. This variation in propensity for treatment among the residents cut the need for dental treatment in half and pointed again to the importance of placing the psychosocial context and potential impact of treatment on an equal footing with physical status. Striking a balance between invasive treatment and supportive psychologic counselling is a challenge in any context, but it is especially difficult amid the many conflicting priorities of LTC and the unavoidable politics of a multidisciplinary health service [24].

Adaptation to cope with disability

Disability is not necessarily a pathologic process; rather, it may be an inevitable part of healthy aging that we will all experience if we live long enough [88]. Successful aging is not a linear process of decline but rather a dynamic, fluctuating, and resilient process of change, both for the worse and for the better, in which individuals adapt to cope with life and maintain a sense of coherence [89]. Typically, this transition is achieved initially by assimilating whatever is to hand to compensate for a perceived loss of self-esteem and identity, followed by a process of accommodation in which activities are modified and expectations reduced [90]. Recognizing the complexity and resilience of health, disability, and quality of life in old age is central to the development and implementation of a successful strategy for managing oral health in LTC facilities.

Oral health and quality of life in long-term care

The concept of quality of life is offered as a guiding beacon to good care on the assumptions that it reflects self-esteem and life-satisfaction and that it has measurable properties that facilitate accountability and quality assurance [91]. It is, nonetheless, a concept laden with cultural values and influenced by personal goals, expectations, standards, and concerns. It is difficult, therefore, to capture quality of life within a narrow response to illness or within the limitations of health care, even by qualifying it as "health-related quality of life" [92]. Quality of life must also be distinguished from the more limited "quality of care" concept associated with medical and nursing care [93]. Caregivers, for example, frequently rate the quality of life of their patients much lower than do the patients themselves [94]. Yet, for all the uncertainty surrounding the concept, it can draw attention to the complexity of life and the undeniable resilience of old age. Ultimately, the concerns dominating oral health care in LTC revolve around the comfort and safety of the residents in the facilities. These concerns pose difficult challenges for dental professionals as they struggle over their own preference for ideal treatment versus practical treatment and over society's preference for autonomy versus beneficence [95]. Although many disagree on what constitutes a reasonable range of oral health care services, a just allocation of resources, and fair financial compensation, society clearly expects a health service that is effective, accessible, available, and affordable. Our social responsibility must lead us to address oral health care from an egalitarian perspective, recognizing that health is a necessary precondition of "equality of opportunity" even in the midst of severe frailty [96]. Appropriate care for frail elders should combine a focus on prevention with a social contract offering curative care with the aim of providing maximum benefit to the least advantaged in society [97].

Future research needs

Much work is needed to resolve the many issues of prevention in the complex environment of LTC facilities and to provide effective curative care for individuals, no matter how frail, who could benefit from comprehensive dental services.

Research is required to identify the characteristics of aging populations who are benefited or disturbed by oral health care. Do oral health factors, such as poor oral hygiene, disturb frail elders or cause premature death? No oral health–related screening method exists that is valid and reliable for use by nurses and care aides, and the methods proposed for examining older adults need further testing to confirm their value as predictors of oral disease and dysfunction.

Caries is very difficult to control and manage in LTC. Can active carious lesions be identified sensitively and specifically from inactive or dormant lesions? What are the physical and psychosocial characteristics of a frail elderly person who is at high risk for caries? Is it possible or desirable to limit the amount of sugar and other cariogenic foods available in nursing homes, and can fluoride or other preventive interventions be used effectively to reduce the risk of caries to a manageable level?

Poor oral hygiene and gingivitis are rampant in nursing homes and appear not to cause much concern to the residents, in contrast to their impact on more independent elders. What degree of plaque accumulation causes physical or psychologic discomfort to frail elders? Does the accumulation change with increasing frailty to the point where general health is compromised? What are the most effective strategies for educating nurses and care aides about oral health and hygiene? Can legislation on oral health care be enforced effectively in an institutional environment with so many conflicting priorities—and are regulations even desirable in societies that emphasize the autonomy of the individual?

LTC facilities need more input from dental personnel, but it is not clear what combination of personnel is needed or what factors influence this combination. How can dental professionals be encouraged to work in LTC facilities? Should dental hygienists be the primary oral health providers in LTC, or are they more effective when dentists provide the initial diagnoses and treatment plans? Dentists are neither comfortable nor confident providing comprehensive restorative treatment in a facility without a fully equipped dental clinic. How can dentists be educated and encouraged to provide this service, and what is the minimum treatment needed to maintain the psychologic and physical comfort (including nutritional health) of a frail resident?

Finally, the widespread interest in quality of life as a measurable outcome of dental disorder and curative intervention needs elaboration beyond the negative focus on oral disadvantage, deprivation, and handicap that currently predominates. How do the complicated and various psychosocial responses of old age help frail elders to cope with oral disability without experiencing abnormality or loss? Is it possible to make the enhancement of the quality of life of elderly LTC patients a central objective of dentistry, by improving our knowledge of the relationship between oral health and frailty and by clarifying the role of dental personnel in this relationship?

References

[1] Kinsella K, Velkoff VA. US Census Bureau, Series P95/01-1. An aging world: 2001. Washington, DC: US Government Printing Office; 2001. Available at: http://www.census.gov/prod/2001pubs/p95-01-1.pdf. Accessed May 8, 2004.

[2] Robine J-M, Mormiche P, Cambois E. Evolution des courbes de survie totale, sans maladie chronique et sans incapacité en France de 1981 à 1991: application d'un modèle de l'OMS. Ann Demogr Hist (Paris) 1996;99–115.

[3] Hill GB, Forbes F, Lindsay J, et al. Life expectancy and dementia in Canada: the Canadian study of health and aging. Chronic Dis Can 1997;18(4):166–7.

[4] Grundy E. Demographics and gerontology: mortality trends among the oldest old. Aging & Society 1997;17:713–25.

[5] Broderick E. Prescribing patterns for nursing home residents in the US. The reality and the vision. Drugs Aging 1997;11(4):255–60.

[6] Rockwood K, Fox RA, Stolee P, et al. Frailty in elderly people: an evolving concept. Can Med Assoc J 1994;150(4):489–95.

[7] Buchner DM, Wagner EH. Preventing frail health. Clin Geriatr Med 1992;8(1):1–17.

[8] McCormick JC, Chulis GS. Growth in residential alternatives to nursing homes: 2001. Health Care Financ Rev 2003;24(4):143–50.

[9] Adult care regulations (Community Care Facilities Act). British Columbia Reg. 536/80. Community Care and Assisted Living Act, SBC. Victoria, British Columbia: Ministry of Health Services, Queen's Printer; 2003. s.47.

[10] Canadian Council on Hospital Accreditation. Standards for accreditation of Canadian long-term care centres. Standard Number 5. Ottawa (ONT): 1985.

[11] Government of British Columbia. Order in Council #1105. Appended and ordered October 1st, 1997 to amend Section 9 of the Adult Care Legislation. Victoria (BC): 1997.

[12] Thai PH, Shuman SK, Davidson GB. Nurses' dental assessments and subsequent care in Minnesota nursing homes. Spec Care Dentist 1997;17(1):13–8.

[13] Call RL, Berkey D, Gordon SR. Compliance with long-term care regulations: advocacy or passive neglect. Gerodontology 1987;3:165–8.

[14] Gift HC, Cherry-Peppers G, Oldakowski RJ. Oral health care in US nursing homes, 1995. Spec Care Dentist 1998;18(6):226–33.

[15] US Department of Health and Human Services. Healthy people 2010 (conference edition, in 2 volumes). Washington, DC: 2000.

[16] MacEntee MI, Weiss R, Waxler-Morrison NE, et al. Factors influencing oral health in Vancouver's long-term care facilities. Community Dent Oral Epidemiol 1987;15(6):314–6.

[17] MacEntee MI, Scully C. Oral disorders and treatment implications in people over 75 years. Community Dent Oral Epidemiol 1988;16(5):271–3.

[18] Berkey DB, Berg RB, Ettinger RL, et al. Research review of oral health status and service use among institutionalized older adults in the United States and Canada. Spec Care Dentist 1991;11(4):131–6.

[19] Lamy M, Mojon P, Kalykakis G, et al. Oral status and nutrition in the institutionalized elderly. J Dent 1999;27(6):443–8.

[20] Hawkins RJ, Main PA, Locker S. Oral health status and treatment needs of Canadian adults aged 85 years and over. Spec Care Dentist 1998;18(4):164–9.

[21] Wyatt CC. Elderly Canadians residing in long-term care hospitals. Part I.. Medical and dental status. J Can Dent Assoc 2002;68(6):353–8.

[22] Wardh I, Andersson L, Sorensen S. Staff attitudes to oral health care: a comparative study of registered nurses, nursing assistants and home care aides. Gerodontology 1997;14(1):28–32.

[23] MacEntee MI, Thorne S, Kazanjian A. Conflicting priorities: oral health in long-term care. Spec Care Dentist 1999;19(4):164–72.

[24] Thorne S, Kazanjian A, MacEntee MI. Oral health in long term care: the implications of organizational culture. J Aging Stud 2001;15:271–83.

[25] Weiss RT, MacEntee MI, Morrison BJ, et al. The influence of social, economic, and professional considerations on services offered by dentists to long-term care residents. J Public Health Dent 1993;53(2):70–5.

[26] MacEntee MI, Waxler-Morrison NE, Morrison BJ, et al. Opinions of dentists on the treatment of elderly patients in long term care facilities. J Public Health Dent 1992;52(4):239–44.

[27] Ablah CR, Pickard RB. Dental hygienists and long-term care. J Dent Hyg 1998;72(2):27–34.

[28] Wood GJ, Mulligan R. Cross-sectional comparison of dental students' knowledge and attitudes before geriatric training: 1984–1999. J Dent Educ 2000;64(11):763–71.

[29] Bryant SR, MacEntee MI, Browne A. Ethical issues encountered by dentists in the care of institutionalized elders. Spec Care Dentist 1995;15(2):79–82.

[30] Besdine RW, Rubenstein LZ, Cassel C. Nursing home residents need physicians' services [editorial]. Ann Intern Med 1994;120(7):616–8.

[31] O'Connor CE, Carr S. Interdisciplinary collaboration between nursing and dental hygiene: clinical care for the elderly. J Gerontol Nurs 1981;7(4):233–5.

[32] Chalmers JM, Levy SM, Buckwalter KC, et al. Factors influencing nurses aides' provision of oral care for nursing facility residents. Spec Care Dentist 1996;16(2):71–9.

[33] Blanco VL, Levy SM, Ettinger RL, et al. Challenges in geriatric oral health research methodology concerning caregivers of cognitively impaired adults. Spec Care Dentist 1997; 17(4):129–32.

[34] Fure S. Ten-year incidence of tooth loss and dental caries in elderly Swedish individuals. Caries Res 2003;37(6):462–9.

[35] MacEntee MI, Clark DC, Glick N. Predictors of caries in old age. Gerodontology 1993; 10(2):90–7.

[36] Johannsen I, Birhed D. Diet and the caries process. In: Thylstrup A, Fejerskov O, editors. Clinical cardiology. Copenhagen (Denmark): Munksgaard; 1994. p. 283–310.

[37] MacEntee MI, Wyatt CCL, McBride B. A longitudinal study of caries and cariogenic bacteria in an elderly population. Community Dent Oral Epidemiol 1990;18(3):149–52.

[38] Stamm JW, Banting DW, Imrey PB. Adult root caries survey of two similar communities with contrasting natural water fluoride levels. J Am Dent Assoc 1990;120(2):143–9.

[39] Baysan A, Whiley RA, Lynch E. Antimicrobial effect of a novel ozone-generating device on micro-organisms associated with primary root carious lesions in vitro. Caries Res 2000;34(6): 498–501.

[40] Banting DW, Papas A, Clark DC, et al. The effectiveness of 10% chlorhexidine varnish treatment on dental caries incidence in adults with dry mouth. Gerodontology 2000;17(2): 67–76.

[41] Saunders RH, Davila E, Hayes AL, et al. The effectiveness of sponge-type intraoral applicators for applying topical fluorides in institutionalized older adults. Spec Care Dentist 1994;14(6):224–8.

[42] Bader JD, Shugars DA, Bonito AJ. A systematic review of selected caries prevention and management methods. Community Dent Oral Epidemiol 2001;29(6):399–411.

[43] Wyatt CCL, MacEntee MI. Caries management for institutionalized elders using fluoride and chlorhexidine mouthrinses. Community Dent Oral Epidemiol 2004;32(1):1–7.

[44] Wyatt CCL, MacEntee MI. Dental caries in chronically disabled elders. Spec Care Dentist 1998;17(6):196–202.

[45] Pearson A, Chalmers J. Oral hygiene care for adults with dementia in residential aged care facilities. Joanna Briggs Institute Reports 2004;2(3):65–113.

[46] MacEntee MI, Silver J, Gibson G, et al. Oral health in a long term care institution equipped with a dental service. Community Dent Oral Epidemiol 1985;13(5):260–3.

[47] US Public Health Service. Surgeon General's report on oral health. Chapter 4. Bethesda (MD): Department of Health and Human Services, NIH, NIDCR; 2000. Available at: http://www.nidcr.nih.gov/sgr/sgrohweb/chap4.htm#dental_caries. Accessed April 9, 2004.

[48] Steele JG, Treasure E, Pitts NB, et al. Total tooth loss in the United Kingdom in 1998 and implications for the future. Br Dent J 2000;189(1):598–603.

[49] Mojon P, Thomason JM, Walls AWG. The impact of falling rates of edentulism. Int J Prosthodont 2004, in press.

[50] Mojon P, MacEntee MI. Discrepancy between need for prosthodontic treatment and complaints in an elderly edentulous population. Community Dent Oral Epidemiol 1992; 20(1):48–52.

[51] Mojon P, MacEntee MI. Estimates of time and propensity for dental treatment among institutionalized elders. Gerodontology 1994;11(2):99–107.

[52] Steele JG, Sheiham A, Marcenes W, et al. Diet and nutrition in Great Britain. Gerodontology 1998;15(2):99–106.

[53] World Health Organization. A review of current recommendations for the organisation of community oral health services in northern and western Europe. Copenhagen (Denmark): World Health Organization (regional office for Europe); 1992.

[54] Van Waas MA, Meeuwissen JH, Meeuwissen R, et al. Oral function in dentate elderly with reduced dentitions. Gerodontology 1993;10(1):40–3.

[55] Sheiham A, Steele JG, Marcenes W, et al. The relationship among dental status, nutrient intake, and nutritional status in older people. J Dent Res 2001;80(2):408–13.

[56] Shimazaki Y, Soh I, Saito T, et al. Influence of dentition status on physical disability, mental impairment and mortality in institutionalised elderly people. J Dent Res 2001; 80(1):340–5.

[57] MacEntee MI, Campbell T. Personal identification using dental prostheses. J Prosthet Dent 1979;41(4):377–80.

[58] Bryant SR, Zarb GA. Outcomes of implant prosthodontic treatment in older adults. J Can Dent Assoc 2002;68(2):97–102.

[59] Feine JS, Carlsson GE, Awad MA, et al. The McGill Consensus Statement on Overdentures. Montreal, Quebec, Canada, May 24–25, 2002. Int J Prosthodont 2002;15(4):413–4.

[60] Walton JN, MacEntee MI, Hanvelt R. A cost analysis of fabricating implant prostheses. Int J Prosthodont 1996;9(3):271–6.

[61] Walton JN, MacEntee MI. A prospective study on the maintenance of implant prostheses in private practice. Int J Prosthodont 1997;10(5):453–8.

[62] MacEntee MI, Hill PM, Wong G, et al. Predicting concerns for oral health among institutionalized elders. J Public Health Dent 1991;51(2):82–91.

[63] Terpenning MS, Taylor GW, Lopatin DE, et al. Aspiration pneumonia: dental and oral risk factors in an older veteran population. J Am Geriatr Soc 2001;49(5):557–63.

[64] Shay K. Infectious complications of dental and periodontal diseases in the elderly population. Clin Infect Dis 2002;34(9):1215–23.

[65] Brown LJ, Brunelle JA, Kingman A. Periodontal status in the United States, 1988–91: prevalence, extent, and demographic variation. J Dent Res 1996;75(Spec Iss):672–83.

[66] Gornitsky M, Paradisi I, Landaverde G, et al. A clinical and microbiological evaluation of denture cleansers for geriatric patients in long-term care institutions. J Can Dent Assoc 2002; 68(1):39–45.

[67] Stafford GD, Arendorf T, Huggett R. The effect of overnight drying and water immersion on candidal colonization and properties of complete dentures. J Dent 1986;14(2):52–6.

[68] Banting DW, Hill SA. Microwave disinfection of dentures for the treatment of oral candidiasis. Spec Care Dentist 2001;21(1):4–8.

[69] National Center for Chronic Disease Prevention and Health Promotion. Guidelines for infection control in dental health-care settings—2003. Available at: http://www.cdc.gov/mmwr/preview/mmwrhtml/rr5217a1.htm. Accessed July 21, 2003.

[70] Apse P, Zarb GA, Schmitt A, et al. The longitudinal effectiveness of osseointegrated dental implants. The Toronto Study: peri-implant mucosal response. Int J Periodontics Restorative Dent 1991;11(2):94–111.

[71] MacEntee MI, Hole R, Stolar E. The significance of the mouth in old age. Soc Sci Med 1997; 45(9):1449–58.

[72] Kayser-Jones J, Bird WF, Paul SM, et al. An instrument to assess the oral health status of nursing home residents. Gerontologist 1995;35(6):814–24.

[73] Bauer JG. The index of ADOH: concept of measuring oral self-care functioning in the elderly. Spec Care Dentist 2001;21:63–7.

[74] MacEntee MI, Wyatt CC. An index of clinical oral disorder in elders (CODE). Gerodontology 1999;16(2):85–96.

[75] Kayser-Jones J, Bird WF, Redford M, et al. Strategies for conducting dental examinations among cognitively impaired nursing home residents. Spec Care Dentist 1996;16(2):46–52.

[76] Lin CY, Jones DB, Godwin K, et al. Oral health assessment by nursing staff of Alzheimer's patients in a long-term-care facility. Spec Care Dentist 1999;19(2):64–71.

[77] Weeks JC, Fiske J. Oral care of people with disability: a qualitative exploration of the views of nursing staff. Gerodontology 1994;11(1):13–7.

[78] Hardy DL, Brangan PP, Darby ML, et al. Self-report of oral health services provided by nurses' aides in nursing homes. J Dent Hyg 1995;69(2):75–82.

[79] Kay EJ, Locker D. Is dental health education effective? A systematic review of current evidence. Community Dent Oral Epidemiol 1996;24(4):231–5.

[80] Frenkel HF, Harvey I, Newcombe RG. Improving oral health in institutionalised elderly people by educating caregivers: a randomised controlled trial. Community Dent Oral Epidemiol 2001;29(4):289–97.

[81] Arvidson-Bufano UB, Blank LW, Yellowitz JA. Nurses' oral health assessments of nursing home residents pre- and post-training: a pilot study. Spec Care Dentist 1996;16(2):58–64.

[82] Paulsson G, Söderfeldt B, Nederfors T, et al. The effect of an oral health education program after three years. Spec Care Dentist 2003;23(2):63–9.

[83] Schou L, Wight C, Clemson N, et al. Oral health promotion for institutionalised elderly. Community Dent Oral Epidemiol 1989;17(1):2–6.

[84] Brown LF. Research in dental health education and health promotion: a review of the literature. Health Educ Q 1994;21(1):83–102.

[85] Käyser AF. How much reduction of the dental arch is functionally acceptable for the ageing patient? Int Dent J 1990;40(3):183–8.

[86] MacEntee MI, Hole R, Stolar E. The significance of the mouth in old age. Soc Sci Med 1997; 45(9):1449–58.

[87] Fiske J, Davis DM, Frances C, et al. The emotional effects of tooth loss in edentulous people. Br Dent J 1998;184(2):90–3.

[88] Bury M. Illness narratives: fact or fiction? Sociol Health Illn 2001;25:263–85.

[89] Rowe JW, Kahn RL. Human aging: usual and successful. Science 1987;237(4811):143–9.

[90] Brandstädter J, Greve W. The aging self: stabilizing and protective processes. Dev Rev 1994; 14:52–80.

[91] Slade G, editor. Measuring oral health and quality of life. Chapel Hill (NC): Department of Dental Ecology, School of Dentistry, University of North Carolina; 1997.

[92] Allison PJ, Locker D, Feine JS. Quality of life: a dynamic construct. Soc Sci Med 1997;45(2): 221–30.

[93] Gentile KM. A review of the literature on interventions and quality of life in the frail elderly. In: Birren JE, Lubben JE, Rowe JC, et al, editors. The concept and measurement of quality of life in the frail elderly. San Diego (CA): Academic Press; 1991. p. 74–88.

[94] Pearlman RA, Uhlmann RF. Quality of life in chronic disease: perceptions of elderly patients. J Gerodontol 1988;43(2):M25–30.

[95] Bryant SR, MacEntee MI, Browne A. Ethical issues encountered by dentists in the care of institutionalized elders. Spec Care Dentist 1995;15(2):79–82.

[96] Dharamsi S, MacEntee MI. Dentistry and distributive justice. Soc Sci Med 2002;55(2): 323–9.

[97] Rawls J. A theory of justice. Cambridge (MA): Harvard University Press; 1971.

ELSEVIER
SAUNDERS

THE DENTAL
CLINICS
OF NORTH AMERICA

Dent Clin N Am 49 (2005) 445–461

Oral Diagnostics for the Geriatric Populations: Current Status and Future Prospects

Yolanda Ann Slaughter, DDS, MPH[a],
Daniel Malamud, PhD[b],*

[a]Department of Preventative and Restorative Sciences, School of Dental Medicine,
University of Pennsylvania, 240 South 40th Street, Philadelphia, PA 19104, USA
[b]Department of Biochemistry, School of Dental Medicine, University of Pennsylvania,
240 South 40th Street, Philadelphia, PA 19104, USA

Because it is a noninvasive technique, there is growing interest in replacing blood with oral-based methods of diagnostics. Oral diagnostics may be used for diagnosis and therapeutic drug monitoring of both oral diseases (eg, caries, periodontal disease, oral lesions, oral cancer) and systemic diseases (eg, infectious diseases, including HIV and AIDS, autoimmune diseases, cancer, and endocrine disorders). Two general approaches to oral diagnostic analyses exist: (1) an oral sample may be collected and sent to a central site for analytic testing or (2) the sampling and analysis may be performed on site, a process referred to as point-of-care diagnostics. For hospitalized patients, laboratory analysis of blood or urine samples is routine; for mobile outpatients and functionally dependent or homebound individuals, point-of-care diagnostics would be a major advance. The benefits of oral sampling as opposed to blood testing include safety (little or no contact with blood), cost-effectiveness, and increased patient compliance, particularly in compromised subjects, such as infants, children, and geriatric subjects. Indeed, whether because of dehydration, sclerosed veins, or limited tolerance to the procedure [1], geriatric patients demonstrate unique difficulties in blood draws.

A number of reviews of saliva-based and other oral-based diagnostics have recently appeared [2–8]; however, none of these has focused on

This work was supported by Grant No. UO1-DE014964 from the National Institutes of Health.

* Corresponding author.
E-mail address: malamud@pobox.upenn.edu (D. Malamud).

applications for the geriatric populations. In the present review and commentary, the authors address both existing techniques and oral-based diagnostics that will be applicable to the aging population in the future. They also highlight those techniques that are uniquely suited to point-of-care applications.

It is well known that most molecules found in blood or plasma also can be detected by sampling the oral cavity. The accuracy of any diagnostic test is defined by its sensitivity, specificity, predictive value, and efficiency [9]. The major issues in developing a successful oral diagnostic test are the sensitivity of the assay and the relationship of the oral level of the analyte to the reference blood levels. Sensitivity is an issue because most molecules in saliva are present at lower levels than those found in blood. Fortunately, advances in amplification and detection technologies now permit analyses at the low concentrations of analyte found in oral samples. The relationship of the oral level to the plasma level, the saliva/plasma (S/P) ratio [10], is relevant when quantitative values are required from the diagnostic test. For a qualitative assay—for example, the presence or absence of antibodies to HIV—the only issue is sensitivity. The oral test must be sensitive enough to detect the lower levels of antibodies found in the oral cavity, but because the HIV diagnosis is "yes or no," the exact amount of antibody present is not required. In contrast, for therapeutic drug monitoring or determining blood alcohol concentration with salivary samples, the S/P ratio must be constant over a range of plasma concentrations if the diagnostic test is to be useful.

Fluids from the oral cavity that can be used for analysis include whole saliva, parotid saliva, submandibular saliva, minor salivary gland secretions, gingival crevicular fluid (GCF), and oral mucosal transudate. A description of these fluids and a summary of methods for their collection have been published in the Guidelines for Saliva Nomenclature and Collection section of the *Annals of the New York Academy of Sciences* [3]. In addition, oral tests may use buccal epithelial cells as a source of DNA [11], oral/pharyngeal swabs for identification of a number of infectious pathogens, a cytobrush for oral cancer detection [12], and volatiles to assess malodor or gastrointestinal dysfunction [13,14]. A new approach to saliva collection that might be particularly useful to homebound or institutionalized geriatric populations is self-collection with the Oracol sponge device (Malvern Medical Developments, Worcestershire, United Kingdom). This device, along with a questionnaire, was mailed to 14,800 individuals in an epidemiologic survey designed to monitor antibodies to infections [15]. Returned samples were successfully tested for antibodies to a number of viral pathogens.

The decision about which type of oral sample to collect will largely depend on the biologic question being asked. In quantitative diagnostics, one can often predict whether the S/P ratio will be constant based on the characteristics of the molecule being analyzed. This is because the mechanism whereby a molecule enters the oral cavity is the major determinant of the S/P ratio. For example, some molecules enter the oral cavity by direct diffusion from the blood, whereas others enter by active transport following tissue damage or by blood contamination of saliva. Unconjugated steroid hormones, such as dehydroepiandrosterone (DHEA), freely cross cell membranes, and thus salivary levels correlate closely with blood levels. However, the conjugated form of this hormone, dehyroepian-drosterone sulfate (DHEAS), does not freely diffuse into saliva. Some reports have demonstrated that DHEA measurements have an acceptable S/P ratio, whereas other reports note that the addition of sulfate impairs the lipid solubility of DHEA and thus the value of the salivary measurement as an index of blood levels of DHEAS [16].

A second factor to consider in the case of steroid hormones is that blood contains both free and protein-bound steroid hormone, whereas saliva contains only free hormone. In blood tests one either measures total hormone (bound plus free) or separates the two forms before assay. In contrast, salivary measurements of steroid hormones only detect free hormone. This limitation could be a positive attribute, because the free hormone concentration is often more relevant to biologic effects. Similar considerations may apply to therapeutic drug monitoring, because blood may contain both free and bound forms of the drug, whereas saliva will typically only contain free drug. The factors that affect the transport of a molecule from blood to saliva include molecular weight, pH, surface charge, hydrophobicity, and protein binding [17]. Some large molecules (eg, albumin) enter saliva as a result of tissue damage, leakage, or blood contamination. Blood contamination can be assessed by monitoring a known marker, such as hemoglobin [18] or transferrin [19]. It is then possible either to discard the contaminated samples or correct for leakage from blood.

Oral diagnostics: lifespan developmental ideas

As the population continues to age and to benefit from advances in managing chronic illnesses, a growing number of persons will fit the paradigm of successful aging [20–23]. This phenomenon will be seen dramatically in the aging baby boomers. The desire to maintain quality of life and good functionality over the lifespan sets the stage for use of oral diagnostics, which may have particular relevance to risk assessment and monitoring of disease onset and severity among various older adult cohorts. As the population continues to change in size and diversity [24], there will necessarily also be changes in the demand for health care delivery among the young-old (65 to 75 years), the old-old (75 to 85 years), and the oldest-old (>85 years) [25–28]. Because increasing functional disabilities affect an individual's ability to seek medical and dental services [29], health care providers should be developing collaborations to provide both oral and general health care, using novel methods that permit multiple tests from easily obtained samples [30]. Health care of the elderly from head to foot is complex and relies on a host of specialists—for example, the physician, dentist, nurse, social worker, physical therapist, and nutritionist. Home-bound and institutionalized elders have good access to medical health care delivery. However, they are often unaware of oral health needs and of the relationship between oral health and general health. The authors believe that the development of new diagnostics for oral and systemic health will enhance communication between dental and medical health care providers and integrate oral health into the overall health care of the individual.

Overview of lifespan developmental issues

Functionally independent older adults

These persons are characterized as living in the community and requiring little to no assistance in their activities of daily living (ADL) [31]. This group constitutes the vast majority (85%) of the older adult population [32] and will increase dramatically as the baby boomers become "senior boomers" [20]. The senior boomers tend to place a high value on health, in part owing to their ability to pay for these services [20]. The senior boomers are characterized as using medical and dental services on a regular basis and as being accustomed to the advances of modern medicine and dentistry [27]. They are expected to continue using health services as they did when they were younger [27]. Because this group is aware of preventive medicine, its members are likely to perceive oral testing as beneficial to their health. Moreover, the senior boomers are expected to engage in behaviors that maintain their health, and oral-based testing may be a strategy for successful aging. Specific testing might assess caries activity, periodontal status, steroid hormone levels that affect postmenopausal bone loss, and possible onset of cancer, diabetes mellitus, or coronary heart disease [22,33–35].

Frail older adults

These persons reside in the community and require assistance in their ADL because of chronic physical, medical, or emotional problems [31]. This group includes homebound older adults, who constitute 10% of the older adult population [32]. The current dental care delivery system is least equipped to meet the needs of these homebound elders [36]. This deficiency is due in part to a dearth of dental providers who have geriatrics training and are willing to provide mobile services, and in part to barriers imposed by Medicare/Medicaid, which excludes dental services to the elderly [24,32,36]. Point-of-care diagnostics could identify systemic conditions or emotional problems that characterize the functional status of this population. The homebound population and its caregivers highly value point-of-care medical services that accommodate their desire to avoid institutionalization [36]. Therefore, the use of oral tests to monitor chronic illnesses that influence the elders' ability to remain at home would be particularly favorable to the caregiver. The medical providers have access to the homebound elders and have developed trusting relationships with the patients and caregivers. The initiation of oral health promotion by the visiting medical provider, by means of oral diagnostic testing, may motivate the homebound elder and the caregiver to view oral health as integral to maintaining general health. In the future, oral tests may include monitoring for nutritional deficiencies, which plays an important role in promoting medical and dental health care. Vitamin and nutrient deficiencies lead to oral signs and symptoms; they also influence resistance to disease and the ability to repair damaged tissues. Common systemic illnesses that affect frail elders, such as diabetes, chronic obstructive pulmonary disease, osteoporosis, and atherosclerotic cardiovascular disease, are well known to be associated with malnutrition [37]. Although point-of-care diagnostics for malnutrition do not yet exist, this is clearly an area for future development.

Functionally dependent older adults

These persons reside in nursing homes and constitute 5% of the older adult population [32]. This population is so impaired by a combination of physical, mental, or emotional problems that its members are unable to maintain their independence [31]. Unlike the frail homebound elders, elderly nursing home residents have well-documented dental care needs, with oral hygiene poor and chronic oral infections prevalent [31,32,36,38,39]. These elders require total assistance with their personal hygiene, and oral hygiene is not a major concern of the overworked, underpaid, and non–dentally educated staff who are responsible for up to 90% of their daily care [38,39]. This barrier to dental care delivery has serious implications for the quality of life and potential for successful aging of residents in long-term care facilities. As in the frail homebound population, the use of oral diagnostics by the nursing staff to identify and monitor disease severity in these patients may reduce the risk of acute exacerbations. A greater benefit to the oral hygiene of nursing home residents is seen when nursing aids receive encouragement from other members of the nursing staff, as opposed to instruction by a dentist or hygienist [38]. In this context, oral diagnostics may be a useful approach to educating and motivating nursing aides to consider daily oral health care essential to overall care. Poor oral hygiene and chronic oral infections have been shown to be associated with aspiration pneumonia and bronchopulmonary infections [40,41]. Specific tests applicable to long-term care residents include evaluation of oral and respiratory infections so that they can be treated either prophylactically or therapeutically.

Demand for dental and medical care: cohort differences in dental care need

The graying of America means that people are living longer; however, demographic transition trends among birth cohorts provide a more specific explanation of the process of population aging. Trends in oral disease patterns have resulted in a dramatic decline in total tooth loss with increasing age; more elders are retaining their natural teeth [42]. In the younger generation of elders, this factor is coupled with positive expectations about retaining and maintaining teeth and maintaining good general health over the lifespan. The oldest generation of elders, by contrast, tends to have ageist views about the possibility of retaining teeth and maintaining good general health. These different attitudes of different older populations present a challenge to the dental profession in meeting their care needs [20,25,43,44].

A clear understanding of the patient's desires and needs is key to the clinical decision-making process and is essential for providing care based on rational health assessments of the growing elder population. Perceived need is the most common reason cited by elders for not seeking medical or dental care services [45]. Therefore, this section's discussion of new diagnostic techniques is guided by an awareness of the different perceptions of health care need and attitudes toward health among different generations of the elderly.

Oldest-old (>85 years)

This cohort has the distinction of being the fastest-growing segment of the elderly population, and its health care needs are also increasing dramatically [27–29]. Historically, most people in this age cohort were totally edentate, and tooth loss was considered an inevitable part of growing old [27]. This attitude was due to a lack of money and to a philosophy of dentistry that was not directed toward saving teeth. The typical dental practice was to have teeth extracted in response to symptoms of tooth pain, so many of the aged over 85 wear complete dentures [27]. Patients in this cohort are more likely to suffer from the effects of chronic diseases, of taking multiple drug regimens to treat these problems, and of not seeking dental services, particularly when they are edentulous. Although root caries and periodontal disease are not as prevalent in this cohort [46–48], other age-prevalent changes relevant to oral diagnostic procedures might be used to promote successful aging in collaboration with medical health care providers [49]. Particular interest is focused on elders who lack dental services and who have Alzheimer's disease, stroke, Parkinson's disease, or oral-motor dysfunction disabilities that impair the ability to perform oral self-care behaviors [50–52]. These persons are more susceptible to the adverse health effects of oral pathogens, salivary dysfunction, and adverse drug interactions [53]. Additionally, oral lesions are common among older adults using dental prosthesis [28]. Health care providers have access to this population, in which noninvasive tests may be particularly beneficial because of its tendency toward inadequate oral hygiene due to combativeness or tremors. Risk assessment on the part of the medical provider may facilitate increasing referrals to the dentist to promote overall health.

Specific tests for this population include therapeutic drug monitoring and health assessments applicable to long-term care residents and the frail homebound.

Old-old (≥75 years)

Most people in this cohort have retained more natural teeth and total tooth loss is less common than in the previous cohort [27,28]. These elders use dental services on a more regular basis than the oldest cohort and have benefited from the philosophy of dentistry that focused more on restorative care [28,29]. This cohort is better educated and more financially secure and has experienced more dental contact for preventive services. Although the presence of teeth is reported to be highly correlated to perceived need in this age group—more so than income or education—the expectation of having complete dentures as a normal part of growing old still prevails in this cohort, as in the oldest one [28]. By contrast with the oldest cohort, the trend toward tooth retention, resulting in increased rates of root caries and periodontal disease, is an issue in this one [28,42,47,48]. Dental health is not generally perceived as important by this cohort, so many have unmet oral health issues that can adversely affect chronic conditions and quality of life. Given that people in this cohort have experienced more frequent dental contacts for reasons other than tooth extraction, and that they routinely sent their children to the dentist [28,29], they may be more amenable to changing their demand for dental care when the change is initiated by the medical provider as a means to preserve their health. Like the oldest cohort, these elders are affected by age-prevalent changes and normative age changes that can benefit from oral diagnostic testing.

Young-old (>65 years)

Most people in this cohort are characterized as retaining more natural teeth and having had more regular dental contacts than previous generations. This so-called "new elderly" had the advantages of more education, more consumable income, and the technological advances of modern dentistry [26,28]. The baby boomers constitute a growing proportion of this cohort. Because they are more aware of the benefits of maintaining good medical and dental health, they may hold the most promise for using new diagnostic methods to track medical and dental conditions. The political and social movements experienced by this cohort were fueled by the desire to take action to advance the public well-being. Likewise, the new elderly will likely continue to access dental and medical services, and they will demand continued technological advances in medicine and dentistry to help them achieve successful aging [20,26,28]. Hence, the use of new oral-based tests by this cohort may help persuade third-party insurers to compensate providers for this service. Additionally, the fact that medical providers can easily use oral diagnostic testing may have an impact on policy makers. More emphasis will be directed toward increasing awareness of the importance of oral health to overall health to compress morbidity and decrease medical costs.

The aforementioned cohorts include subsets of persons identified as being low income, members of minority groups, or persons with special needs. These vulnerable elders (including the frail homebound and nursing home residents) have less than ideal access to dental care services compared with their counterparts in the general population [30,54–57]. The opportunity exists for dental providers to build community partnerships on a local level with aging networks that target these underserved groups, such as senior centers, residential care centers, and mental health centers. Oral diagnostics could be incorporated into these community-based programs and provide point-of-care services in a familiar setting. This approach could increase awareness of the relationships between oral and systemic health among the community-dwelling vulnerable elders and could increase the standard of care in residential facilities for special needs elders. Thus, oral diagnostics may serve to decrease health disparities among underserved groups. Other conditions of importance to low-income elders include diagnostics for toxic materials, including heavy metals, because these elders often live in areas that are more exposed to environmental hazards.

Specific applications of oral-based diagnostic tests

Caries

Because a number of factors contribute to caries formation, including host genetic factors, presence of bacterial pathogens, and nutrition, tests that monitor these three factors may prove useful in predicting caries activity. Classic microbial sampling and culture techniques for dental pathogens are widely used. A sample is collected on a swab or paper point and sent in appropriate transfer media to a microbiologic test site. Samples are cultured for approximately 48 hours, and typically the results are sent directly to the clinician to help guide treatment planning. These types of assays can be used for both cariogenic and periodontal organisms, although there is some question about the impact of such testing on subsequent treatment options. A simpler diagnostic system uses test strips to identify either *Streptococcus mutans* or *Lactobacilli* (Dentocult strips, Orion Diagnostica, Finland). The strips are exposed to the oral tissue and then incubated for 48 hours; a colorometric analysis is used to identify the presence of *S mutans* or *Lactobacilli*. Perhaps more relevant to point-of-care diagnostics, several investigators are developing polymerase chain-reaction and microarray-based assays that may be used to identify oral pathogens rapidly [58,59]. The approach uses a miniaturized detection system, sometimes referred to as lab-on-a-chip, which would amplify the signal and give a positive or negative result on site. Rapid test results lead to prompt dental and medical decision-making.

An alternative approach to predicting caries susceptibility is to monitor oral pH or buffer capacity. Because demineralization of the tooth is accelerated in an acid environment, salivary pH and the ability of saliva to buffer bacterial acid production are likely to be related to caries activity. Subjects with high buffer capacity have an increased ability to resist caries formation. Buffer capacity can be assessed quickly with Dentobuff strips (Orion Diagnostica, Finland); this assessment may be useful for identifying individuals who need to be monitored more closely or given additional nutritional counseling and other preventive measures.

Saliva also contains a large number of proteins that help control bacterial colonization, by influencing the balance between bacterial clearance from the oral cavity and adherence to oral tissues [60]. Several recent reviews address this topic [61,62]. Ideally, one would have a single marker that correlates with actual or potential caries activity. One such possibility is suggested by research from the Denny laboratory [63]. Their studies suggest a relationship between the *S mutans* titer in the oral cavity and the concentration of MG2, the low molecular weight mucin present in whole and submandibular saliva [64]. In a study of 24 subjects aged 65 to 82, elevated titers of *S mutans* were associated with decreased levels of MG2. Previous reports from this group had demonstrated that mucin concentration decreases with aging [65]. A rapid test for MG2 in the oral cavity that is amenable to point-of-care diagnosis appears to be feasible and could facilitate identification of elder individuals who are at an increased risk for caries formation.

Periodontal diseases

Advances in the diagnosis of periodontal diseases have focused on new microbiologic methods for detecting periodontal pathogens and on various techniques to monitor the host response to gingival inflammation. As noted earlier for caries diagnostic tests, traditional methods of identifying periodontal pathogens rely on oral sampling followed by bacterial culturing at remote laboratory sites. Newer approaches are using a variety of molecular approaches, which could be adapted to point-of-care diagnostics. In terms of assessing the host responses to periodontal disease, both saliva and GCF tests have been used. Although GCF testing may be valuable, it requires a dental professional to obtain the sample, whereas saliva-based tests could be performed by relatives, care-givers, or even by the functionally independent individual. Analytes that may be useful for monitoring periodontal diseases have recently been reviewed [66–68] and include lactoferrin, collagenase, lysozyme, prostaglandin E2 (PGE2), proinflammatory cytokines, and markers of cell death such as aspartate aminotransferase. To date, no single marker appears to correlate specifically with the presence or extent of periodontal disease, but a constellation of markers may prove to be useful. Another issue raised by oral-based testing for both caries and periodontal disease is the need to educate and encourage the dental professional to support these tests. Some of the geriatric cohorts described earlier may provide this incentive and facilitate controlled clinical trials.

Antibodies/infectious diseases

One of the most successful applications of oral-based diagnostics is the use of an oral sample (saliva or mucosal transudate) to detect antibodies to HIV and a wide range of other infectious agents [69–71]. In general, ductal saliva contains mostly secretory IgA (sIgA), whereas whole saliva and mucosal transudates contain both IgA and IgG antibodies. Crevicular fluid generally has the highest level of immunoglobulins, but difficulties in collection of GCF limit its usefulness. Notably, salivary levels of IgA appear to increase with age [72], suggesting that detection may be easier in a geriatric population. Numerous studies have reported the use of oral fluids for detection of antibodies to a wide range of bacterial, viral, and fungal pathogens, and it is reasonable to predict that if the fluids are a useful source of these antibodies, any antibody can be detected. Because levels of antibody in oral samples are lower than those in blood, more sensitive assays are required. A second generation of sensitive immunoassays using polymerase chain reaction or time-resolved fluorescence may prove particularly valuable for use with oral specimens [73].

Saliva and other oral fluids can also be used to detect antibodies associated with autoimmune diseases. In Sjögren syndrome, for example, there are numerous reports of studies tracking anti–SS-A (anti-Ro) and anti–SS-B (anti-La) antibodies (see [74] for a recent review). In addition, autoantibodies against M3 muscarinic acetylcholine receptors are closely correlated with decreased salivary flow and salivary lysozyme levels [75], suggesting that this may be another useful marker for diagnosing Sjögren syndrome. It has also been reported that salivary antimitochondrial antibodies are associated with primary biliary cirrhosis [76], a disease with increasing prevalence in postmenopausal women.

Therapeutic drug monitoring

One of the major concerns of health care workers managing geriatric clients is therapeutic drug monitoring. One issue in this area is adherence to the prescribed drug regimen: patients may forget, lose track of, or purposely "overdose" on their prescription drugs ("if a little is good, more must be better"). In some cases, the consequences are insignificant, but in many cases the therapeutic window is small, and serious adverse events can result from too little or too much of the prescribed drug.

A large body of literature addresses the use of oral samples for detecting and quantizing the drugs of abuse (eg, ethanol, opiates, cannabis, cocaine, amphetamine) as a noninvasive point-of-care diagnostic [77–79]. In general, these studies have demonstrated that oral testing is as accurate as blood or urine testing, and it is possible to distinguish drugs of abuse from legal drugs (eg, codeine or benzodiazepines). The therapeutics most widely studied with oral tests include anticonvulsants (phenytoin, carbamazepine, and pheno-barbital), cotinine as a measure of tobacco smoke exposure, theophylline, and lithium. Although all these drugs demonstrated acceptable S/P ratios, there appears to be no incentive to develop these as marketable tests, probably because of the perceived modest market size for such diagnostics.

More recently, oral samples have been used to monitor the hormone melatonin [80], the epilepsy drug lamotrigine [81], schizophrenia therapeutics such as clozapine [82], and the anti-HIV drug nevirapine [83]. In all these cases, oral drug levels were correlated with blood or urine levels; however, none of these has been developed as a commercial test. In cases where the patient is hospitalized and blood is routinely collected, there is no incentive to use an oral test for the drug. However, the geriatric population may be an ideal cohort for oral diagnostics, creating an impetus for commercial development.

Cancer

A large body of information exists on saliva-based diagnostics for oral cancer. These studies include antibodies to the common tumor suppressor p53, associated with squamous cell carcinoma of the oral cavity [84,85]. Extraction of DNA from saliva revealed mutations in p53 that were much higher in samples from oral squamous cell carcinoma (5/8, 62%) than in healthy salivary samples (5/27, 18%), suggesting that specific mutations could be used as a molecular marker [86]. In addition, microsatellite analysis using salivary DNA has been used for molecular analysis of tumorigenesis in head and neck carcinoma [87]. Although these changes can be detected by isolating DNA from saliva samples, brushing of the lesion may increase the sensitivity of these assays [88]. Streckfus et al [89] have reported that a number of tumor markers (CA15-3, c-erb-2, EGF receptor, and p53) can be detected in the saliva of women with breast cancer. If confirmed, these findings would provide great impetus for the development of screening tests for breast and perhaps other tumors. The cancer markers just described are compatible with point-of-care diagnostics.

A summary of lifespan developmental stages and age cohorts, as related to relevant oral diagnostics, is presented in Tables 1 and 2.

Future possibilities for oral-based diagnostics

In a number of cases, oral-based tests have demonstrated that a particular analyte can be monitored, but approved commercial tests are not yet available—this is the case, for instance, with monitoring steroid hormone levels. Reports also exist of defensin-1 in saliva associated with oral

Table 1
Oral diagnostics: lifespan developmental stages related to functional status

Functional status	Characteristics	Health care need	Oral diagnostics
Functionally independent older adults	Community-residing; no assistance with ADL	Increasing medical and dental care need with aging baby boomers	Diabetes mellitus, coronary heart disease, cancer, caries/periodontal tests, therapeutic drug monitoring
Frail older adults	Community-residing; assistance with ADL; include homebound	Dental care needs unknown; value point-of-care medical services	Nutritional deficiencies, autoimmune diseases, infectious diseases, dementia, Parkinson's
Functionally dependent older adults	Nursing home residents	Poor oral hygiene and chronic oral infections	Oral and respiratory infections, cancer

inflammation [90] and oral carcinoma [91], C-reactive protein associated with periodontal disease [92], and salivary endothelin associated with chronic heart failure [93]. In addition, there are factors for which oral testing would clearly be useful, but no test yet exists, such as prostate-specific antigen (PSA), vitamin and other micronutrients, and markers for arteriosclerosis, Alzheimer's disease, and Parkinson's disease. One of the potential advantages of point-of-care oral-based diagnostics is the capacity to monitor changes over time, instead of relying on a single determination. For example, it appears that the rate of change in PSA levels may be more

Table 2
Oral diagnostics: lifespan developmental stages related to age cohort

Age cohort	Health care need	Demand for health care	Oral diagnostics
Oldest-old (85 y and older)	Susceptible to health effects from oral pathogens, salivary dysfunction, drug interactions	Increased medical use; little dental contact; most edentate	Therapeutic drug monitoring, autoimmune diseases, nutritional deficiencies, infectious diseases
Old-old (75 y and older)		Increased medical use; more regular dental contact; total tooth loss less common	
Young-old (65 y and older)	Modeling successful aging; more knowledgeable about benefits of maintaining medical and dental health	Regular medical and dental contact; retained more natural teeth	Caries activity, periodontal status, steroid hormone levels, cancer, autoimmune diseases

important in predicting prostate cancer than a single reading. Such might also be the case for markers of inflammation, coronary heart disease, and arteriosclerosis. As more oral tests become approved and as health care providers and health management organizations recognize the potential for such tests, it is likely that efforts will be directed to the identification of markers that can monitor or predict disease.

The National Institutes for Dental and Craniofacial Research have issued a request for applications to identify and develop new oral-based diagnostics (Development of Technologies for Saliva/Oral Fluid Based Diagnostics RFA: RFA-DE-02-002) and have funded seven research projects. Some of these are likely to result in novel detection systems that include point-of-care diagnostics.

With the characterization of the saliva proteome, also supported by NIDCR (The Salivary Proteome: Catalogue Of Salivary Secretory Components RFA: RFA-DE-04-007), a complete catalogue of all salivary proteins will be available, facilitating future studies to correlate specific proteins with specific stages in the aging process. Likewise, the determination and cataloging of all the metabolic small molecules in the oral cavity, referred to as the metabolome, will provide a benchmark for determining specific alterations in these molecules throughout the aging process. It is possible to envision an in-dwelling sensor with capabilities for continuously transmitting data on the levels of proteins, small molecules, and hormones in the oral cavity. Indeed, a number of companies are currently developing biochips that could carry out this type of measurement.

References

[1] McKenna D, Niles SA. Venipuncture: an adjunct to home care services for older adults. Geriatr Nurs (Minneap) 1995;16:208–11.
[2] Malamud D. Saliva as a diagnostic fluid: second now to blood? BMJ 1992;305:207–8.
[3] Malamud D, Tabak L. Saliva as a diagnostic fluid. Ann N Y Acad Sci 1993;694.
[4] Slavkin HS. Toward molecularly based diagnoses for the oral cavity. J Am Dent Assoc 1998; 129:1138–43.
[5] Kefalides PT. Saliva research leads to new diagnostic tools and therapeutic options. Ann Intern Med 1999;131:991–2.
[6] Lawrence HP. Salivary markers of systemic disease: noninvasive diagnosis of disease and monitoring of general health. J Can Dent Assoc 2002;68:170–4.
[7] Streckfus CF, Bigler LR. Saliva as a diagnostic fluid. Oral Dis 2002;8:69–76.
[8] Kaufman E, Lamster IB. The diagnostic applications of saliva: a review. Crit Rev Oral Biol Med 2002;12:197–212.
[9] Galen RS, Gambino SR. The predictive value and efficiency of medical diagnoses. New York: Wiley; 1975.
[10] Siegal IA. The role of saliva in drug monitoring. In: Malamud D, Tabak L, editors. Saliva as a diagnostic fluid. Ann N Y Acad Sci 1993;694:86–90.
[11] Lamey PJ, Nolan A, Follett EA, et al. Anti-HIV antibody in saliva: an assessment of the role of components of saliva, testing methodologies and collection systems. J Oral Pathol Med 1996;25:104–7.

[12] Jones AC, Pink FE, Sandow PL, et al. The Cytobrush Plus cell collector in oral cytology. Oral Surg Oral Med Oral Pathol 1994;77:95–9.

[13] Touyz LZ. Oral malodor—a review. J Can Dent Assoc 1993;59:607–10.

[14] Turner AP, Magan N. Electronic noses and disease diagnostics. Nat Rev Microbiol 2004;2: 161–6.

[15] Morris-Cunnington MC, Edmunds WJ, Miller E, et al. A novel method of oral fluid collection to monitor immunity to common viral infections. Epidemiol Infect 2004;132: 35–42.

[16] Vining RF, McGinley RA. Transport of steroid from blood to saliva. In: Read GF, Riad-Fahmy D, Walker RF, et al, editors. Immunoassays of steroids in saliva. Cardiff (UK): Alpha Omega Publishing; 1982. p. 56–63.

[17] Jusko WJ, Milsap RL. Pharmacokinetic principles of drug distribution in saliva. In: Malamud D, Tabak L, editors. Saliva as a diagnostic fluid. Ann N Y Acad Sci 1993; 694:36–47.

[18] Piazza M, Chirianni A, Picciotto L, et al. Blood in saliva of patients with acquired immunodeficiency syndrome: possible implications of the disease. J Med Virol 1994;42: 38–41.

[19] Schwartz EB, Granger DA. Transferrin enzyme immunoassay for quantitative monitoring of blood contamination in saliva. Clin Chem 2004;50:654–6.

[20] Kiyak HA. Successful aging: implications for health promotion. J Public Health Dent 2000; 60(4):276–81.

[21] Slavkin H. Maturity and oral health: live longer and better. J Am Dent Assoc 2000;131: 805–8.

[22] Ship JA, Chavez EM. Management of systemic diseases and chronic impairments in older adults: oral health considerations. Gen Dent 2000;48(5):555–65.

[23] Miller CS, Epstein JB, Hall EH, et al. Changing oral care needs in the United States: the continuing need for oral medicine. Oral Surg Oral Med Oral Pathol Oral Radiol Endod 2001; 91:34–44.

[24] Berkey D, Berg R. Geriatric oral health issues in the United States. Int Dent J 2001;51(3): 254–64.

[25] Ettinger RL. The unique oral health needs of an aging population. Dent Clin North Am 1997;41(4):633–49.

[26] Ettinger RL, Beck JD. The new elderly: what can the dental profession expect? Geriatr Dent 1982;2(2):62–9.

[27] Ettinger RL. Cohort differences among aging populations: a challenge for the dental profession. Spec Care Dentist 1993;13(1):19–26.

[28] Berkey DB, Berg RG, Ettinger RL, et al. The old-old dental patient. The challenge of clinical decision-making. J Am Dent Assoc 1996;127:321–32.

[29] Ettinger RL, Mulligan R. The future of dental care for the elderly population. CDA J 1999; 27(9):687–92.

[30] US Department of Health and Human Services. Oral health in America: a report of the Surgeon General. Rockville (MD): US Department of Health and Human Services, National Institute of Dental and Craniofacial Research, National Institutes of Health; 2000.

[31] Shay K. Identifying the needs of the elderly patient. The Geriatric Dental Assessment. Practical considerations in special patient care. Dent Clin North Am 1994;38(3):499–523.

[32] Neissen LC, Gibson G. Aging and oral health for the 21st century. Gen Dent 2000;48(5): 544–9.

[33] Jeffcoat MK, Lewis CE, Reddy MS, et al. Post-menopausal bone loss and its relationship to oral bone loss. Periodontology 2000 2000;23:94–102.

[34] Yellowitz JA, Horowitz AM, Drury TF, et al. Survey of US dentists' knowledge and opinions about oral pharyngeal cancer. J Am Dent Assoc 2000;131:653–60.

[35] Ship JA. Geriatric oral medicine. Alpha Omegan 2001;92(2):44–51.

[36] Strayer M. Oral health care for homebound and institutional elderly. CDA J 1999;27(9): 703–8.

[37] Saunders MJ. Nutrition and oral health in the elderly. Dent Clin North Am 1997;41(4): 681–98.

[38] MacEntee MI. Oral care for successful aging in long-term care. J Public Health Dent 2000; 60(4):326–9.

[39] Ellis AG. Geriatric dentistry in long-term care facilities: current status and future implications. Spec Care Dentist 1999;19(3):139–42.

[40] Taylor GW, Loesche WJ, Terpenning MS. Impact of oral diseases on systemic health in the elderly: diabetes mellitus and aspiration pneumonia. J Public Health Dent 2000;60(4): 313–20.

[41] Scannapieco FA, Mylotte JM. Relationship between periodontal disease and bacterial pneumonia. J Periodontol 1996;67(Suppl 10):1114–22.

[42] Marcus SE, Drury TF, Brown LJ, et al. Tooth retention and tooth loss in the permanent dentition of adults: United States 1988–91. J Dent Res 1996;75(Spec Iss):684–95.

[43] Gilbert GH. "Ageism" in dental care delivery. J Am Dent Assoc 1989;118:545–8.

[44] Dolan TA, McNaughton CA, Davidson SN, et al. Patient age and general dentists' treatment decisions. Spec Care Dentist 1992;12(1):15–20.

[45] Kiyak HA. Impact of patients' and dentists' attitudes on older persons' use of dental services. Gerodontics 1988;4:331–5.

[46] Meskin L, Berg R. Impact of older adults on private dental practices, 1988–1998. J Am Dent Assoc 2000;131:1188–95.

[47] Brown LJ, Brunelle JA, Kingman A. Periodontal status in the United States, 1988–91: prevalence, extent and demographic variation. J Dent Res 1996;75(Spec Iss):6726–83.

[48] Winn DM, Brunelle JA, Selwitz RH, et al. Coronal and root caries in the dentition of adults in the United States, 1988–1991. J Dent Res 1996;75(Spec Iss):642–51.

[49] Shay K. Restorative considerations in the dental treatment of the older patient. Gen Dent 2000;48(5):550–4.

[50] Ghezzi EM, Ship JA. Dementia and oral health. Oral Surg Oral Med Oral Pathol Oral Radiol Endod 2000;89:2–5.

[51] Chavez EM, Ship JA. Sensory and motor deficits in the elderly: impact on oral health. J Public Health Dent 2000;60(4):141–6.

[52] Alexander RE, Gage TW. Parkinson's disease: an update for dentists. Gen Dent 2000;48(5): 572–80.

[53] Heft MW, Mariotti AJ. Geriatric pharmacology. Dent Clin North Am 2002;46:869–85.

[54] Kiyak HA, Persson RE, Persson GR. Influences on the perceptions of and responses to periodontal disease among older adults. Periodontology 2000 1998;16:34–43.

[55] Ronis DL, Lang WP, Antonakos CL, et al. Preventive oral health behaviors among African American and white adults in Detroit. J Public Health Dent 1998;58:234–40.

[56] Jones JA, Fedele DJ, Bolden AJ, et al. Gains in dental care not shared by minority elders. J Public Health Dent 1994;54:39–46.

[57] Glassman P, Miller CE. Preventing dental disease for people with special needs: the need for practical preventive protocols for use in community settings. Spec Care Dentist 2003;23(5): 165–7.

[58] Hoshino T, Kawaguchi M, Shimizu N, et al. PCR detection and identification of oral streptococci in saliva samples using gtf genes. Diagn Microbial Infect Dis 2004;48:195–9.

[59] Stahl D. High-throughput techniques for analysing complex bacterial communities. Adv Exp Med Biol 2004;547:5–17.

[60] Rosan B, Appelbaum B, Golub E, et al. Enhanced saliva-mediated bacterial aggregation and decreased bacterial adhesion in caries-resistant versus caries-susceptible individuals. Infect Immunol 1982;38:1056–9.

[61] Nieuw Amerongen AV, Bolscher JGM, Veerman ECI. Salivary proteins: protective and diagnostic value in cariology? Caries Res 2004;38:247–53.

[62] Rudney JD, Hickey KL, Ji Z. Cumulative correlations of lysozyme, lactoferrin, peroxidase, sIgA, amylase, and total protein concentrations with adherence to microplates coated with human saliva. J Dent Res 1999;78:759–68.

[63] Baughan LW, Robertello FJ, Sarrett DC, et al. Salivary mucin is related to oral *S. mutans* in elderly people. Oral Microbiol Immunol 2000;15:10–4.

[64] Denny PC, Denny PA, Klauser DK, et al. Age-related changes in mucins from whole saliva. J Dent Res 1991;70:1320–7.

[65] Navazesh M, Mulligan RA, Kipnis V, et al. Comparison of whole saliva flow rates and mucin concentrations in health Caucasian young and aged adults. J Dent Res 1992;71:1275–8.

[66] Kaufman E, Lamster IB. Analysis of saliva for periodontal diagnosis: a review. J Clin Periodontol 2000;27:453–65.

[67] Ozmeric N. Advances in periodontal disease markers. Clin Chim Acta 2004;343:1–16.

[68] Jentsch H, Sievert Y, Gocke R. Lactoferrin and other markers from gingival crevicular fluid and saliva before and after periodontal treatment. J Clin Periodontol 2004;31:511–4.

[69] Granstrom GP, Askelof P, Granstrom M. Specific immunoglobulin A to Bordetella pertusis antigens in mucosal secretion for rapid diagnosis of whooping cough. J Clin Microbiol 1988; 26:869–74.

[70] Wienholt MG, Erbling R, Bennetts RW, et al. Detection of antibodies to Helicobacter pylori using oral specimens. Ann N Y Acad Sci 1993;694:340–2.

[71] Hodinka RL, Nagahunmugam T, Malamud D. Detection of human immunodeficiency virus antibodies in oral fluids. Clin Diagn Lab Immunol 1998;5:419–26.

[72] Childers NK, Greenleaf C, Li F, et al. Effect of age on immunoglobulin. A subclass distribution in human parotid saliva. Oral Microbiol Immunol 2003;18:298–301.

[73] McKie A, Vyse A, Maple C. Novel methods for the detection of microbial antibodies in oral fluids. Lancet Infect Dis 2002;2:18–24.

[74] Nikitakis NG, Rivera H, Lariccia C, et al. Primary Sjögren syndrome in childhood: report of a case and review of the literature. Oral Surg Oral Med Oral Pathol Oral Radiol Endod 2003; 96:42–7.

[75] Berra A, Sterin-Borda L, Bacman S, et al. Role of salivary IgA in the pathogenesis of Sjögren's syndrome. Clin Immunol 2002;104:49–57.

[76] Ikuno N, Mackay IR, Jois J, et al. Antimitochondrial autoantibodies in saliva and sera from patients with primary biliary cirrhosis. J Gastroenterol Hepatol 2001;16:1390–4.

[77] Cone EJ, Presley L, Lehrer M, et al. Oral fluid testing for drugs of abuse: positive prevalence rates by Intercept immunoassay screening and GC-MS-MS confirmation and suggested cutoff concentrations. J Anal Toxicol 2002;26:541–6.

[78] Bennett GA, Davies E, Thomas P. Is oral fluid analysis as accurate as urinalysis in detecting drug use in a treatment setting? Drug Alcohol Depend 2003;72:265–9.

[79] Niedbala RS, Feindt H, Kardos K, et al. Detection of analytes by immunoassay using up-converting phosphor technology. Anal Biochem 2001;293:22–30.

[80] Gooneratne NS, Metlay JP, Guo W, et al. The validity and feasibility of saliva melatonin assessment in the elderly. J Pineal Res 2003;34:88–94.

[81] Ryan M, Grim SA, Miles MV, et al. Correlation of lamotrigine concentrations between serum and saliva. Pharmacotherapy 2003;23:1550–7.

[82] Dumortier G, Lochu A, Zerrouk A, et al. Whole saliva and plasma levels of clozapine and dimethylclozapine. J Clin Pharm Ther 1998;23:35–40.

[83] Van Heeswijk RP, Veldkamp AI, Mulder JW, et al. Saliva as an alternative body fluid for therapeutic drug monitoring of the nonnucleoside reverse transcription inhibitor nevaripine. Ther Drug Monit 2001;23:255–8.

[84] Tavassoli M, Brunel N, Mahher R, et al. P53 antibodies in the saliva of patients with squamous cell carcinoma of the oral cavity. Int J Cancer 1998;78:390–1.

[85] Warnakulasuriya S, Soussi T, Maher R, et al. Expression of p53 in oral squamous cell carcinoma is associated with the presence of IgG and IgA p53 autoantibodies in sera and saliva of the patients. J Pathol 2000;192:52–7.

[86] Liao PH, Chang VC, Huang MF, et al. Mutations of p53 gene codon 63 in saliva as a molecular marker for oral squamous cell carcinomas. Oral Oncol 2000;36:272–6.

[87] El-Naggar AK, Mao L, Staerkel G, et al. Genetic heterogeneity in saliva from patients with oral squamous carcinomas. Implications in molecular diagnosis and screening. J Mol Diagn 2001;3:164–9.

[88] Nunes DN, Kowalski LP, Simpson AJ. Detection of oral and oropharyngeal cancer by microsatellite analysis in mouth washes and lesion brushings. Oral Oncol 2000;36:525–8.

[89] Streckfus C, Bigler L, Tucci M, et al. A preliminary study of CA15-3, cerbB-2, epidermal growth factor receptor, cathepsin-D, and p53 in saliva among women with breast cancer. Cancer Invest 2000;18:101–9.

[90] Mizukawa N, Sugiyama K, Ueno T, et al. Levels of human defensin-1, an antimicrobial peptide in saliva of patients with oral inflammation. Oral Surg Oral Med Oral Pathol Oral Radiol Endod 1999;87:539–43.

[91] Ganz T, Selsted ME, Szklarek D, et al. Defensins: natural peptide antibiotics of human neutrophils. J Clin Invest 1985;76:1427–35.

[92] Pederson ED, Stank SR, Whitener SJ, et al. Salivary levels of alpha 2–macroglobulin, alpha 1–antitrypsin, C-reactive protein, cathepsin G and catalase in humans with or without destructive periodontal disease. Arch Oral Biol 1995;40:1151–5.

[93] Denver R, Tzanidis A, Martin P, et al. Salivary endothelin concentrations in the assessment of chronic heart failure. Lancet 2000;355:468–9.

THE DENTAL
CLINICS
OF NORTH AMERICA

Dent Clin N Am 49 (2005) 463–484

Osteoporosis: Diagnostic Testing, Interpretation, and Correlations with Oral Health—Implications for Dentistry

Roseann Mulligan, DDS, MS[a,b,*], Stephen Sobel, DDS[a]

[a]University of Southern California, School of Dentistry, 925 West 34th Street,
Los Angeles, CA 90089-0641, USA
[b]University of Southern California, School of Gerontology, 3715 McClintock Avenue,
Los Angeles, CA 90089-0191, USA

Osteoporosis is a condition of the skeleton that is characterized by compromised bone strength and predisposition to an increased risk of fracture. It is the most prevalent metabolic bone disease in this country. Osteopenia describes a condition of bone mass that is lower than normal but not severe enough to be considered osteoporotic. In the third National Health and Nutrition Examination Survey (NHANES III, 1988 to 1994), bone mineral density tests of the femur were completed for the first time [1]. According to the World Health Organization's (WHO) recommended criteria for osteoporosis and reduced bone mineral density (BMD), 56% of women 50 years of age and older had a reduced level of bone density, with 16% of these meeting the criteria for osteoporosis, whereas 18% of men demonstrated reduced BMD (Fig. 1) [1]. Using these data, it is estimated that more than 10 million Americans over the age of 50 have osteoporosis, including 7.8 million women and 2.3 million men; another 33.6 million over the age of 50 have low bone mass and hence are at risk for osteoporosis [2].

Increasing age is clearly a factor in osteoporosis, with an age-related BMD loss of 1% to 2% per year. Women in their 80s have a 10 times greater risk of being osteoporotic than women in their 50s (Fig. 2) [1]. Some racial and ethnic groups are more vulnerable to this condition, with non-Hispanic whites and Asians being at higher risk than Mexican Americans or non-Hispanic blacks [2]. Osteoporosis also is more prevalent in individuals with

---

* Corresponding author. University of Southern California, School of Dentistry, 925 West 34th Street, Room 4338, Los Angeles, CA 90089-0641.

E-mail address: mulligan@usc.edu (R. Mulligan).

0011-8532/05/$ - see front matter © 2005 Elsevier Inc. All rights reserved.
doi:10.1016/j.cden.2004.10.005
dental.theclinics.com

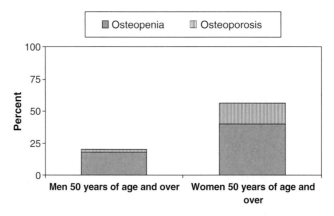

Fig. 1. Prevalence of low femur bone density in the United States as reflected in NHANES III, 1988–94. (*From* Department of Health and Human Services. Centers for Disease Control and Prevention. National Center for Health Statistics. Osteoporosis. National Health and Nutrition Survey (NHANES III). Available at: http://www.cdc.gov/nchs/data/nhanes/databriefs/osteoporosis.pdf. Accessed July 3, 2004.)

less than a 12th-grade education than it is in those who had a 12th-grade education or higher [3].

Overall, osteoporosis results in 1.5 million fractures per year: 700,000 are vertebral; 250,000 are wrist fractures; 300,000 are located in a variety of sites; and 300,000 are in the hip, resulting in a mortality of 25% [4]. One of every two women and one of every four men will have a fracture related to osteoporosis. By the year 2001, the direct medical costs of osteoporotic fractures came to $17 billion for the year [4], and the annual costs are expected to continue to rise.

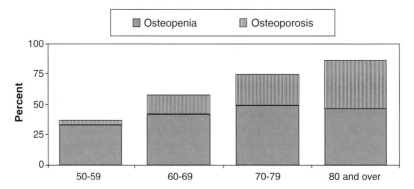

Fig. 2. Prevalence of low femur bone density in older women in the United States as reflected in NHANES III, 1988–94. (*From* Department of Health and Human Services. Centers for Disease Control and Prevention. National Center for Health Statistics. Osteoporosis. National Health and Nutrition Survey (NHANES III). Available at: http://www.cdc.gov/nchs/data/nhanes/databriefs/osteoporosis.pdf. Accessed July 3, 2004.)

Osteoporosis is likely to become an even larger contributor to morbidity and mortality as the population of the United States continues to gray. By the year 2000, 12.4% of the population was 65 years of age or older, amounting to 35 million people. It is projected that by the year 2020, 20% of the population, or 54 million people, will be over 65.

Data from the National Health Interview Surveys of 1983 and 1993 also demonstrate that more adults are retaining teeth, with disparities in the number of teeth remaining based on age and race or ethnicity [5]. More and more elderly people are seeking care from oral health providers to maintain oral health. What are the issues linking oral health and osteoporosis? We know that prevention is a key to avoiding osteoporosis. How might dentists be engaged in a preventive role? Is osteoporosis detectable with dental radiography techniques? Do the current medications for osteoporosis have an impact on oral health? Are they likely to cause adverse interactions with medications that are typically used in dental practices? Do these medications also play a positive role in maintaining the density of the mandible and maxilla? Should dentists be prescribing medications for osteoporosis to maintain the health of the oral facial complex? Should fluoride usage be prescribed for the elderly, not only to decrease caries but to strengthen bone? All these questions are addressed in this article.

The nature of osteoporosis

Osteoporosis is a result of low bone mass and weakening of the microarchitecture of the bone that results in an increased risk of fracture [6]. Different types of bone undergo different changes. For example, cortical bone loss occurs mainly from the endosteal surfaces, resulting in enlarged marrow cavities, whereas affected bone of the vertebrae shows disruption in the trabecular network as a result of weakening of the horizontal supporting struts [7]. Bone is in a continuous state of resorption and deposition [8]. During aging, the balance between these activities is disturbed, resulting in a negative bone mass change. Bone strength can be predicted by bone mass and bone quality changes. Bone mass frequently is measured by dual energy x-ray absorptiometry (DEXA). Bone quality, which is related to microarchitecture, mineralization, and mechanical properties, cannot be assessed by DEXA technology and hence is assessed using invasive techniques such as density fractionation, microradiography, and microhardness testing or noninvasive techniques such as back scattered electron imaging. Typically, screening protocols call for the use of DEXA measurements [9].

Measuring bone density using dual energy x-ray absorptiometry

DEXA is a noninvasive and painless way to measure bone mass or density. Although a number of sites can be measured (eg, spine, femur, radius, calcaneus), chosen primarily for their high incidence of osteoporotic fractures, there is some debate as to the best site for predicting osteoporosis. The best way to assess BMD at a particular site is to measure that area directly, rather than having a measurement at another site serve as a proxy for the region of interest [10].

The purposes of BMD testing are multiple. This testing can detect low bone density before a fracture occurs, confirm a diagnosis of osteoporosis, predict the possibility of future fractures, determine the rate of bone loss, and monitor the effects of treatment [4].

DEXA results are reported as t-scores and z-scores. The t-scores are comparisons of the patient's BMD with a young population's peak reference value, whereas the z-scores are comparisons of the patient's BMD with a population's age-matched reference value, allowing a comparison with the patient's peer group [11]. Using WHO criteria, a patient with a BMD score greater than a 2.5 standard deviation (SD) below the young average peak bone mass (the t-score) is considered osteoporotic. If the BMD score is between 1 SD and 2.5 SD below the t-score, the patient is considered osteopenic [12]. Cautions should be applied to the use of these reference values for those who are not white women, such as Asian women and men of all ethnic and racial groups.

The goal for those with a diagnosis of osteopenia is to prevent the onset of osteoporosis by modifying behavior, increasing nutrient intake, or taking medications. Those with osteoporosis need to engage in treatments that provide active therapy to prevent further bone loss and foster bone deposition. The National Osteoporosis Foundation recommends treatment for those with a BMD t-score greater than a −2 when there are no risk factors or greater than −1.5 when there are coexisting risk factors or a prior vertebral or hip fracture has occurred [13].

Risk factors

Risk factors for osteoporosis include female gender, white or Asian ancestry, thinness or small frame (<127 lbs), advanced age, a family history of osteoporosis, postmenopausal condition, hyperthyroidism, certain medications (eg, corticosteroids, anticonvulsants), a diet low in calcium, an inactive life-style, cigarette smoking, excessive use of alcohol, and low testosterone. In addition to the risk factors for osteoporosis, fracture risk is increased by poor bone quality and higher rates of falling in the elderly [2,4,6,14].

Screening for risk

In an effort to predict reliably who is at risk for osteoporosis, so that diagnostic tests (typically DEXA studies) may be performed and warranted preventive or therapeutic measures initiated, there have been attempts to develop risk assessment protocols. Michaelsson et al [15] suggested using body weight alone, whereas others have developed screening questionnaires. A three-item Osteoporosis Risk Assessment Instrument (ORAI) based on age, weight, and current estrogen usage demonstrated a sensitivity of 93.3% and a specificity of 46.4% for accurately assessing women who have low BMD [16]. The Simple Calculated Osteoporosis Risk Estimation (SCORE) uses age, race, history of rheumatoid arthritis, history of nontraumatic fracture after age 45, estrogen use, and weight [17]. It has similar sensitivity and specificity outcomes to the ORAI [18]. The goal of these instruments is to help identify women in the population who are at the greatest risk for osteoporosis and have them undergo DEXA examinations, without referring all women for such a diagnostic work-up.

Prevention of osteoporosis

Interventions to prevent osteoporosis should include physical conditioning that incorporates muscle strengthening and coordination activities, nutrients, reduction of behavioral risk factors, and pharmacotherapies [7]. Osteoporosis can be prevented by weight-bearing exercise (eg, walking, hiking, jogging, stair-climbing, weight training, tennis, dancing), a diet rich in calcium and vitamin D [19], healthy habits, with no smoking or excessive alcohol intake [20], bone density testing, the use of certain medications that promote bone health, and minimal use of medications such as glucocorticoids and anticonvulsants, which contribute to bone loss [21].

Diet and nutrients

The American diet is highly deficient in calcium, with elderly females consuming approximately one third of the daily recommended intake and males consuming about one half. The need for increased calcium intake with aging is recognized. Increases in the daily dose of calcium are recommended, in view of the less efficient absorption of this mineral from the intestinal tract of older individuals [8]. Decreases in 25-hydroxy vitamin D also occur with age [22]. Vitamin D is important because it facilitates intestinal calcium absorption and new bone formation. Vitamin D is made in the skin, but aging is accompanied by a decrease in skin composition and thickness [23] that affects vitamin D production. In some parts of the country, because of climate, the elderly are less likely to be outside where they have sun exposure; the same is true of those who are institutionalized [24]. Therefore, their diets must be supplemented. Patients on calcium supplements are less than half as likely to lose teeth as those who are not, according to work by Krall et al [25], although once a patient stops taking calcium and vitamin D the odds for tooth loss immediately increase. Even with a daily intake of 1000 mg of calcium alone, the odds of losing teeth are half those of people who do not take calcium—a result that does not obtain from taking vitamin D alone [25].

High sodium and animal protein intake increases urinary calcium loss and thus is a significant risk factor for osteoporotic fracture. However, when there is low protein intake, a condition referred to as protein-calorie malnutrition occurs. This deficiency stimulates bone resorption and impedes bone formation directly and indirectly through a reduction in serum insulin-like growth factor I [21]. Additionally, the malnourished are more likely to fall and, having less padding over their bones to absorb falls, have a greater risk for fracture. Deficiency of vitamin K and excessive intake of vitamin A also may contribute to osteoporotic fractures [21].

Caffeine and nicotine effects

Smoking has been recognized as a significant risk factor for osteoporosis [26]. Direct effects are due to nicotine's action on bone cells and possibly to the effects of cadmium. Indirect effects include decreased intestinal calcium absorption, changes to vitamin D or in the metabolism of multiple hormones in the body, and the decreased body weight and physical activity that are typically seen in smokers compared with nonsmokers [27]. Studies have shown smoking to have a negative effect on men and women, with some studies showing a greater effect in older men. Increased bone loss due to smoking may be slowed or reversed once smoking has stopped [27]. Hip fractures have been shown to be strongly associated with smoking [28], as have vertebral fractures [29] and fractures at other sites [30].

High caffeine consumption has been implicated as a cause of low BMD. Although some investigators have conjectured that this finding is due to a reduced consumption of milk by avid coffee drinkers [31], others have demonstrated that increased caffeine intake (greater than an equivalent of 18 ounces of brewed coffee per day) accelerates spinal bone loss in elderly women [32].

Although drinking alcohol is associated with lower bone density in pre-menopausal women, moderate amounts of alcohol seem to have a protective effect in postmenopausal woman [33,34]. Heavy alcohol consumption is, however, a strong risk factor for osteoporosis, being associated with impaired osteoblast function that results in suppression of bone turn-over and formation [35]. The inhibition of calcium absorption is another direct effect of heavy alcohol use with negative indirect effects related to the reduction of testosterone levels in men, deterioration of liver function, and protein-calorie malnutrition [36]. The threshold for adverse effects of alcohol is lower in women than in men. Of course, inebriation from alcohol overuse also greatly increases the risk of falling, with a fracture being the potential result.

The contribution of hormone replacement therapy

Bone loss in adults typically occurs in two distinct portions of the lifespan: one period of bone loss occurs around menopause (type I or high turn-over osteoporosis) and another relates to advancing old age (type II or low bone turn-over osteoporosis) [37]. Although men are protected from the former, the osteoporosis of old age is of concern to them as well. Overall decreases in bone mass are greater in women than in men, because at the time of menopause substantial decreases in estrogen levels occur in women. These decreases in estrogen strongly correlate to increased bone loss. When estrogen levels are replaced through hormone replacement therapy (HRT), a protective effect on bone loss and a reduced fracture incidence are demonstrated [38]. Similar decreases do not occur in men. The positive effect of HRT in maintaining BMD only occurs while the hormone is being administered; as a result, no upper age limit has been established for stopping this therapy [38].

It has been conjectured that HRT might also protect bones in the maxilla or mandible. A 7-year longitudinal study by Krall et al [39] followed 189 women who had no HRT. A definite decrease in bone density related to tooth loss was found, even while controlling for menopause and smoking. August et al [40] performed a chart review of people who had received implants in the maxilla (n = 761) and in the mandible (n = 652) and then grouped the subjects by estrogen status: postmenopausal without HRT, postmenopausal with HRT, premenopausal, men younger than 50 years, and men aged 50 or older. No statistically significant differences between groups or sites were found; however, there were also no controls over variables (eg, smoking) that might have confounded the effect.

This study and others demonstrate the need to develop specific measurement protocols that control for confounding factors and to use a longitudinal approach to answer questions about the effect of osteoporosis on oral skeletal findings [41].

Pharmacotherapies for osteoporosis

Several pharmacologic agents, with various mechanisms of action, are used in the treatment of osteoporosis. Calcitonin and bisphosphonates inhibit bone resorption. Selective estrogen-receptor modulators (SERMs) have an estrogen-like effect on the skeleton. Whichever medication regimen is prescribed, the key to successful treatment and prevention is adequate concomitant intake of calcium and vitamin D.

Calcium and vitamin D

Supplemental calcium (in addition to that achieved in the diet) and vitamin D are safe and cost-effective measures to prevent bone loss resulting from osteoporosis [21]. These nutrients should be recommended in the dosages applicable for the age of the patient (Table 1). The recommended dosage for individuals aged 65 and over is 1500 mg of calcium and 600 to 800 IU of vitamin D per day [19].

Table 1
Optimal calcium requirements as recommended by the National Institutes of Health Consensus
Development Conference, June 6–8, 1994

Group	Optimal daily intake (in mg of calcium)
Infant	
Birth–6 mo	400
6 mo–1 y	600
Children	
1–5 y	800
6–10 y	800–1200
Adolescents/Young adults	
11–24 y	1200–1500
Men	
25–65 y	1000
Over 65 y	1500
Women	
25–50 y	1000
Over 50 y (postmenopausal)	1500
On estrogens	1000
Not on estrogens	1500
Over 65 y	1500
Pregnant and nursing	1200–1500

From Optimal calcium intake. NIH Consensus Statement Online 1994 (June 6–8); 12(4):
1–31. Available at: http://consenus.nih.gov/cons/097/097_statement.htm. Accessed August 11,
2004.

Bisphosphonates

The bisphosphonates are so named because they have a phosphate-carbon-phosphate bond. This class of medication induces a shift in mineralization. Binding strongly to hydroxyapatite crystals, they inhibit bone resorption, thus reducing the rate of bone turn-over. They also are potent inhibitors of osteoclasts and reduce the rate at which new bone remodeling units are formed, thereby reducing the depth of resorption. Overall, the result is to produce a positive bone balance at individual remodeling units, which increases bone mass. Alendronate (Fosamax) and risedronate (Actonel) are the two bisphosphonates that are approved by the US Food and Drug Administration for use in the treatment of osteoporosis.

The recommended dose of alendronate (the first bisphosphonate to be approved for osteoporosis, in 1995) for the treatment of osteoporosis is 10 mg per day and may be taken as one weekly dose of 70 mg. The dose recommended for prevention of osteoporosis is half that amount [42]. Instructions for taking alendronate are very specific in terms of timing, posture, and use of water. Following these instructions is crucial for absorption of the medication and avoidance of side effects. This medication must be taken on an empty stomach on rising in the morning with 6 to 8 ounces of water. The patient must stay upright for 30 minutes after taking the medication and not consume any food or other medications during that time. Alendronate is contraindicated in patients with esophageal emptying delays, such as stricture or achalasia, and it can cause esophagitis, a potentially serious side effect in a small percentage of patients. Alendronate may also cause taste alterations [42].

Risedronate differs from alendronate in its chemical structure, but the instructions for its use are similar to and as specific as those for alendronate. The recommended dose for risedronate is 5 mg per day, and it may be taken as a weekly dose of 35 mg [42]. The dose is the same for both treatment and prevention of osteoporosis. Risedronate may increase the gastrointestinal side effects of aspirin and nonsteroidal anti-inflammatory drugs. Patients taking either of these bisphosphonates should be taking supplemental calcium and vitamin D if their dietary intake is inadequate [42].

Etidronate was the first bisphosphonate studied for treatment of osteoporosis [43]. Although it is approved for use in Paget's disease and hypercalcemia of malignancy, it is not approved for treatment of osteoporosis in the United States. However, because it is inexpensive and well tolerated, it is sometimes used "off label" in the United States for osteoporotic patients who cannot tolerate other bisphosphonates [43]. Etidronate is available in tablet form and as an injectable. Parenteral administration may cause taste alterations [42].

Similarly, pamidronate is an injectable bisphosphonate approved for Paget's disease and hypercalcemia of malignancy but not approved for osteoporosis in the United States. It too is sometimes used "off label" for patients who cannot tolerate or absorb oral bisphosphonates [43].

Zoledronate, the most potent bisphosphonate, is available for intravenous administration only. It is approved for hypercalcemia of malignancy and metastatic bone disease and is only used in oncology units and hospitals [42]. Trials to evaluate the antifracture effect of intravenous zoledronate are under way. The potential side effect of significance to dentistry is oral candidiasis [42].

Ibandronate is another bisphosphonate that is in clinical trials for the treatment of osteoporosis.

Selective estrogen-receptor modulators

Tamoxifen, an effective agent in the treatment of breast cancer that has an antiestrogenic effect on breast tissue, has been observed to have an estrogen-like effect on the skeleton [44]. Although tamoxifen is not approved for the treatment of osteoporosis, this serves to demonstrate that an estrogen-like compound that binds with high affinity to the estrogen receptor could have either estrogen agonist or antagonist activity, according to the type of estrogen-responsive tissue. The clinical interest in SERMs is linked to the limitations of HRT. The potential risks of long-term HRT include uterine bleeding and breast cancer [44].

Raloxifene, the first of the second-generation SERMs to be available worldwide for the treatment of osteoporosis, prevents postmenopausal bone loss and reduces the incidence of vertebral fractures and new breast cancer cases in osteoporotic patients without stimulating the endometrium [44]. The observations that estrogens may play a crucial role in the bone metabolism of men and that SERMs prevent bone loss and produce prostatic atrophy in orchidectomized male rats [45] suggest that SERMs may be useful for the treatment of elderly men.

Tibolone, a synthetic steroid, acts on the estrogen, progesterone, and androgen receptors. It does this directly or indirectly through its metabolites, with different patterns depending on the target tissue. It prevents bone loss in early and late postmenopausal women [46,47], reduces menopausal symptoms, has a neutral effect on the endometrium [44], and does not induce breast tenderness. Tibolone has been used in the United Kingdom, Mexico, and South America for the last 20 years. It is still in trials in the United States, where there is some concern that the risk of breast cancer may be linked to its use [48].

Calcitonin

Calcitonin is a polypeptide hormone that regulates calcium and bone metabolism. It has direct renal effects and direct actions on the gastrointestinal tract and is associated with a decreased rate of bone resorption, resorptive activity, and number of osteoclasts [49]. Originally it was available only as an injectable. Now a nasal spray preparation of salmon calcitonin is available [50], with a dose of 200 IU administered intranasally in alternate nostrils daily. Side effects of the nasal spray are minimal, the most significant one being rhinitis. Potential side effects of dental significance are dry mouth and metallic taste, but these are infrequent. Administration of calcitonin should always be accompanied by optimum calcium and vitamin D intake. Calcitonin, when injected, has been found to have an analgesic effect on bone pain associated with acute vertebral fracture, Paget's disease, and bony metastasis. It may play a role in the management of acute vertebral fractures by decreasing analgesic dependence and immobilization. It does not appear to have a role in reduction of hip fracture risk [14].

Fluoride

Fluoride has been shown to have a high affinity for bone and has been used in the past to prevent skeletal fractures because of its ability to stimulate osteoblastic activity without increasing bone resorption [51]. Although the positive effects of drinking fluoridated water on rates of dental caries are well documented, the same cannot be said for water fluoridation and BMD. Early studies were in conflict, leading some scientists to conclude that fluoride ingestion increases fractures, whereas others came to the opposite conclusions. These contradictions appear to be explained by the fact that fluoride's outcome on BMD is dose-dependent. A lower level of fluoride in water (eg, about 1 mg/L) has a positive effect on bone strength; however, higher levels of community water fluoridation correlate with an increased level of fractures [51].

Studies that examine the use of fluoride as a preventive or therapeutic treatment for osteoporosis on an individual basis have typically enrolled too few people to be conclusive, although trends for increased BMD of the lumbar spine when fluoride and HRT are given together have been found [51]. Intermittent fluoride dosing (ie, 15 mg/d, 3-month continuous dosing followed by a 1-month holiday) for a study duration of 3 years demonstrated a significant increase at all lumbar, femur, and radial sites measured [52].

A meta-analysis demonstrating no protective effects was recently completed on studies using fluoride treatment for osteoporosis [13]. However, such an analysis is difficult, because of the number of different fluoride compounds and other covariables (eg, HRT, calcium, vitamin D) that were part of the protocols of the various studies.

The low cost of fluoride compared with many of the other pharmacologic interventions available for prevention or treatment of osteoporosis and the narrow range of benefit versus detriment that fluoride appears capable of causing on the skeleton clearly point to the need for continuing study in this area.

Anabolic agents

It was observed as early as the 1930s that parathyroid hormone (PTH) could have an anabolic action on the skeleton [53]. Teriparatide (rhPTH[1–34]), an anabolic therapy for osteoporosis, has recently been approved by the US Food and Drug Administration. It stimulates new bone formation on trabecular and cortical (periosteal or endosteal) bone surfaces by preferential stimulation of osteoblastic activity over osteoclastic activity. Another anabolic agent, strontium ranelate, provides an alternative approach. The strontium ion appears to be incorporated into the hydroxyapatite crystalline structure and binds to its surface. This process prevents osteoclasts from resorbing bone efficiently, but it does not impede the ability of osteoblasts to make new bone [53].

Statins

Other approaches include the development of statins that reportedly increase bone formation in growing rodents [54] and could also modulate osteoclast function through their actions on the mevalonate pathway. The applicability of current statins is thought to be limited, because they are optimized for liver rather than bone uptake [53].

Oral effects of medications for the treatment of osteoporosis

A number of scientists are examining the bone-growth enhancing effects of the bisphosphonates in improving the outcomes of oral treatments. For example, in an experimental effort to improve bone deposition around dental implants, dogs [55] with hydroxyapatite-coated and titanium machine–polished (TMP) dental implants coated with alendronate were compared with controls. The findings indicated that locally applied alendronate increases the early bone formation rate around implants and results in greater bone-to-implant contact with TMP implants. These findings resemble those of Denissen et al [56], who performed similar experiments in goats and found alveolar bone deposition around bisphosphonate-complexed hydroxyapatite implants in the animals. In another study, rats who received systemic alendronate before and after surgery demonstrated less alveolar bone loss and better fibrosis and collagen bundle formation after mucoperiosteal flap surgery than those receiving saline [57].

Not all findings concerning the bisphosphonates and dental or oral health have been salutary. Bisphosphonates are known to cause mucosal erosions. In a case report published by Demerjian et al [58], a 54-year-old man being treated with alendronate for steroid-induced osteoporosis presented with severe oral ulcers. Instead of swallowing the alendronate, the patient was sucking on the tablets. It is important to instruct patients in the proper use of the bisphosphonate medications to reduce the potential for these harmful outcomes.

Another negative finding was published by Ruggiero et al [59], who reviewed 63 cases of osteonecrosis of the jaw. The common clinical feature was chronic bisphosphonate therapy of 56 patients who had received intravenous bisphosphonates for at least 1 year and 7 patients who were on long-term oral bisphosphonates. The typical lesions were exposed bone or nonhealing extraction sites. Most of the lesions did not respond to conservative debridement and antibiotics and had to be surgically corrected. The findings suggest that oral health care providers should monitor patients on chronic bisphosphonate therapy for this potential complication.

Positive findings emerged from a study of nonosteoporotic patients with periodontitis on a 6-month regimen of alendronate. These subjects demonstrated an increase in maxillary and mandibular bone density over controls, suggesting that alendronate could play the role of an adjunct to conventional periodontal therapy [60]. Reddy et al [61] reviewed the bisphosphonate literature and concluded that there is a potential role for these medications in periodontitis management.

Osteoporosis in men

Osteoporosis in men was scarcely recognized 20 years ago, and to this day it is not generally perceived as a significant problem among men. Although the risk is one third of that for women, when osteoporosis occurs in men the mortality is greater. Fortunately, the health professions now recognize the scope of the problem, and osteoporosis in men is the subject of much active research. However, in view of the limited information available, recommendations come from assumptions based on the current understanding of bone biology and pathophysiology and from the much larger experience with osteoporotic women.

Several factors contribute to the etiology of osteoporosis in men. Over half of men with osteoporosis have secondary osteoporosis, which is associated with other medical conditions, medications, or life-style factors that result in bone loss and fragility. The most important of these are alcohol abuse, glucocorticoid excess, and hypogonadism. A significant portion of men with osteoporosis have idiopathic disease [62].

Several possible contributors have been identified in osteoporosis of unknown origin. Most prominent among them are genetic factors, given that bone density and fracture risk are heritable. Hypogonadism is associated with low BMD, and an important cause of severe hypogonadism is androgen deprivation therapy for prostate cancer.

Life-style factors that contribute to the risk of osteoporosis in men include inadequate nutrition, physical inactivity, and tobacco use.

The recommendations for prevention of osteoporosis in men are similar to those for women [62]. In early life, proper nutrition and exercise have positive effects on bone mass. These principles and avoidance of life-style factors known to be associated with bone loss remain important throughout life. It was previously recommended that men over age 50 have a daily intake of 1200 mg of calcium. That recommendation has been changed to 1500 mg per day of calcium [18], and the suggested intake of vitamin D ranges from 600 IU/d to 800 IU/d [19].

Treatment of osteoporosis in men, as in women, is an extension of prevention. Adequate intake of calcium and vitamin D and appropriate physical activity are essential. Secondary causes of osteoporosis should be identified and treated. The indications for pharmacologic therapies are similar for men and women. Alendronate and PTH are effective in idiopathic osteoporosis, regardless of age or gonadal function. Alendronate and risedronate are effective in glucocorticoid-induced osteoporosis [62]. Testosterone replacement therapy increases BMD in men with hypogonadism, but the effect on fracture risk is unknown. This therapy is appropriate for management of the hypogonadal syndrome, but men with osteoporosis and low testosterone levels should be treated with a bisphosphonate or PTH [62].

Estradiol levels in men better predict BMD than do testosterone levels. BMD for men cannot be extrapolated from that of women; gender-specific reference databases must be used. Androgen therapy may increase BMD in men with hypogonadism or low testosterone, but no data on BMD effects of testosterone therapy exist. As in women, bisphosphonate therapy has been shown to increase BMD in men with osteoporosis.

Evidence supports the beneficial effect of administration of a thiazide diuretic on bone mass, rates of bone loss, and hip fracture risk in men. Other diuretics do not seem to impart the same benefits. The mechanism for the positive effect is not clear, but it has been hypothesized to stem from the decreased excretion of calcium in the urine [63].

Osteoporosis and oral health

Because the lifetime osteoporotic fracture rate is so high for the elderly, investigators remain interested in the possibility of detecting osteoporosis in the maxilla or mandible during routine dental diagnostic procedures. These studies have been criticized for being preliminary and cross-sectional in nature and for not controlling for many variables, such as HRT and smoking, thus leaving unresolved the question of whether mandibular bone density was indicative of systemic bone density [64,65].

If osteoporosis does manifest in the mandible or maxilla, some investigators hypothesize that its presence should have a significant effect on oral findings. Initial work in this area using DEXA technology was accomplished by von Wowern et al [66,67]. Subsequently, others have studied edentulous mandibles using DEXA techniques [68–71]. In general, older women are at greater risk for bone mineral content (BMC) loss of the mandible than are older men. For edentulous individuals, the height of the residual ridge correlates with both the total body calcium and the mandibular BMD [72].

In an effort to continue this line of inquiry, some investigators have attempted to use as measurements of osteoporosis the diagnostic clinical data that are routinely collected in the dental office. For example, Jonasson et al [73] attempted to detect osteoporosis by using periapical radiographs of mandibular alveolar bone as well as dental cast measurements, which were then correlated with DEXA of the forearm. Significant correlations between the BMD of the forearm and alveolar bone (ratio = 0.46; $P < 0.001$) were found; however, interdental cast bone measurements did not correlate, possibly because they did not take into consideration the size of the patient. The authors also found that a gross impression of coarseness of trabeculation, as seen on dental periapical radiographs, significantly correlated to BMD of the forearm (ratio = 0.62), with dense trabeculation being a strong indicator of high BMD, sparse trabeculation a predictor of low BMD, and radiographs demonstrating intermediate trabeculation less obviously correlated.

Although recent literature reveals more interest in systemic disease as a factor in alveolar bone loss, functional factors also may be relevant, because it is well known that tension on bone caused by muscles is a positive force. Therefore, some theorize that it is important to replace missing dentition with implants to ensure function by duplicating loading and thus ensuring bone density [74,75].

Because residual ridge resorption is a common and incapacitating problem in edentulous mandibles, several studies suggest a correlation between ridge resorption and osteoporosis [72,76]. Some examinations through radiologic studies indicate that the mineral density of the cortex and the bone mass in the mandible may be correlated with skeletal bone density. However, in edentulous mandibles, most resorption occurs in the alveolar process without much change to the basal portion. It is here that the bone mass of the mandible is greatest and the functional stresses of mastication may positively impact bone density. These considerations lead some to conclude that routine radiologic measurements are unlikely to be able to assess the effect of osteoporosis on alveolar resorption [77].

Southard et al [78] pointed out that studies that measured BMD were in the posterior alveolar process and examined thick cortical bone, rather than in the anterior mandible and maxillary bone, which have more trabecular bone. Given that areas with trabecular bone are more sensitive to the measurement and detection of bone density decline and that this type of bone is subject to bone loss before cortical bone, these researchers hypothesized that the anterior mandible and maxilla are the regions of interest and that these sites should be the focus for further measurements and comparisons. They therefore designed a protocol specifically to determine whether there were correlations between the BMD of the anterior maxillary and mandibular alveolar processes and that of the spine, hip, or radius in healthy women and found significant correlations of maxillary bone density with all other sites. The lumbar spine, hip trochanter, and mandibular alveolar process correlated at a moderate level (ratio > 0.50). Weaker correlations were found for the radius and total hip measurement (ratio < 0.40), whereas the mandibular readings correlated with the maxilla and no other site [78]. The authors conjectured that the lack of mandibular BMD correlation with other skeletal sites may be due to the presence of mandibular tori or other unexplained causes and that, therefore, this area requires additional study with larger sample sizes.

Implants and osteoporosis

Because dental implants are viewed as viable therapies for our increasingly older population, a number of investigators have focused on their success and longevity in patients with diagnosed or undiagnosed osteoporosis. Becker et al [79] searched for a relationship between osteoporosis in other bones and the maxilla or mandible to predict implant success. Using a strong (case-controlled) study design, they assessed each patient using (1) peripheral DEXA (pDEXA) bone measurements at the distal and proximal radius and ulna, (2) classification of bone quality and quantity at the time of implant placement by visualization, and (3) a questionnaire collecting data variables that could potentially affect the outcome. They found no association between the pDEXA scores at the radius and ulna and the risk for implant failure, yet the visual assessment of bone quality made at the time of placement showed a moderate relationship to implant failure [79]. Becker et al [79] also compared thin cortical bone sites with placements where the cortical bone was thicker or where there was compact bone; as expected, the latter had 2.3 times greater success. These findings demonstrate that the pDEXAs of the radius or ulna are not predictive of implant failure and do not perform better than visual assessments. They do not rule out the possibility that DEXAs of other bones of the skeleton may be better prognosticators of implant success than the pDEXAs and visual assessments.

Looking at the same issue, van Steenberghe et al [80] described a prospective study of 399 consecutive patients with a mean age of 50 and an age range of 15 to 80 years. They concluded that a diagnosis of systemic osteoporosis did not lead to early implant failure; however, poorer bone quality, as determined by radiographic or CT scans, and a preoperative tactile assessment did have a negative impact on survival. Friberg et al [81] followed 13 implant patients who were referred for a medical work-up subsequent to implant placement as a result of the detection of risk factors for osteoporosis. During the mean follow-up period of 3 years and 4 months, the overall success rate for implant placement in these patients with confirmed osteoporosis or osteopenia was 97.1% when an adapted bone site preparation technique and extended healing times were employed.

Future study directions

To determine whether there is an oral effect on all the systemic treatments for osteoporosis, special jaw bone scanners are needed. Likewise, gender-related normative scales for BMC and BMD need to be developed. But especially desirable is the development of a way to study the magnitude of the site-specific effect of treatment.

Von Wowern et al reviewed 115 papers on clinical findings concerning systemic and jaw osteoporosis [82]. The future directions they discuss include especially constructed jaw bone scanners and development of a corresponding gender-related set of normal BMC and BMD values for young adults, as in other sites of the skeleton. The authors suggest that site-specific measurement modalities need to be developed to determine whether treatments such as bisphosphonate medications have positive or negative effects on the BMC and BMD of the jaw bones and their various components in a variety of situations, such as edentulous patients, overdenture conditions, and peri-implant sites [82].

Preventive actions for dentists

The ground for the development of osteoporosis is laid early. Educating teenagers, girls in particular, about consuming enough calcium to achieve their peak bone mass will do much to build bone mass and decrease risk for osteoporosis as aging occurs [83]. Dentists should know the recommended doses of calcium and vitamin D for each age group (see Table 1) and provide guidance about the optimal use of these products to their patients [19,84]. Because dentists see their patients on a regular basis throughout the life span, typically twice a year, they are in a unique position to promote healthy behaviors. The following are suggested strategies that dentists can easily pursue in their practices to promote systemic bone health, thus potentially promoting a healthier oral facial complex.

Osteoporosis-preventive strategies for the dental office

Diet analysis

Diet analysis is routinely done for caries risk assessment. At the same time, the dentist can evaluate whether a patient's diet is appropriate or needs modification for the prevention of osteoporosis.

Life-style considerations

Diets that are good for teeth are generally good for overall health. Dental professionals encourage smokers to quit and advise patients with un-diagnosed but suspected systemic conditions to be evaluated by the appropriate health care provider. If a patient is perceived to be at risk (eg, postmenopausal women), it is appropriate to recommend evaluation. Exercise does not prevent or treat caries or periodontal disease, but exercise can always be recommended as part of the health promotion picture.

Medication misuse

Patients who take prescription or over-the-counter medications arbi-trarily or inappropriately should be encouraged to reconsider and consult the physician if appropriate, and patients who have discontinued their medications without consulting the physician must be encouraged to reconsider.

Standard of care and risk assessment

Taking a medical history is standard. By being thorough and following up on positive findings, the dentist may find clues to potential problems that are not initially obvious. Using one of the short risk assessment questionnaires previously discussed in this paper, dentists can detect who is at risk for osteoporosis and refer these patients to the physician for DEXA screening and treatment strategies.

Common sense

The dental environment (eg, office, clinic) should be set up to minimize the risk of falls. Patient positioning must be done with patient safety and comfort in mind. Adequate head and neck support is essential.

Research and the future

If well-designed, controlled studies find indicators of osteoporosis in dental radiographs, dentists will be among the first health care providers with an opportunity to recognize disease activity and to recommend evaluation for osteoporosis. As a profession, we are already among the first to refer patients to rule out (or rule in) hypertension and other cardiovascular conditions, diabetes, allergic diseases, and neoplasms, among many other possible problems.

Summary

Osteoporosis, the most prevalent metabolic bone disease in the United States, affects over 10 million people, results in over 1.5 million fractures per year, and imposes medical costs of $17 billion per year. Impressive technological advances in the noninvasive evaluation of bone mass and bone density aid in the assessment and diagnosis of osteoporosis. Preventive strategies, although effective, often are initiated too late to offset damage. The medical approach to treatment remains predominantly pharmacologic, with various classes of medication regimens available. Regardless of the medication indicated for a particular patient, the key to prevention and treatment remains adequate intake of calcium and vitamin D throughout life.

Dentistry is in a position to aid in the prevention and evaluation of osteoporosis, primarily by doing what has always been appropriate practice: taking a thorough history, analyzing diet, and encouraging healthy life-style behaviors. If future research finds more evidence of the correlation between the bones of the orofacial complex and systemic osteoporosis, or if it confirms positive outcomes of bisphosphonate therapy for periodontitis treatment and the enhancement of osseointegration of implants, dentists may find themselves prescribing such drugs.

References

[1] Department of Health and Human Services. Centers for Disease Control and Prevention. National Center for Health Statistics. Osteoporosis. National Health and Nutrition Survey (NHANES III). Available at: http://www.cdc.gov/nchs/data/nhanes/databriefs/osteoporosis.pdf. Accessed July 3, 2004.

[2] Anonymous. Report of the Surgeon General's workshop on osteoporosis and bone health. Washington, DC, December 12–13, 2002. Department of Health and Human Services. Available at: http://www.surgeongeneral.gov/topics/bonehealth/workshop_report/pdf/Summary_Final.PDF. Accessed July 24, 2004.

[3] Centers for Disease Control. Osteoporosis among estrogen-deficient women—US. MMWR Morbid Mortal Wkly Rep 1998;47(45):969–72.

[4] National Osteoporosis Foundation. Disease statistics. Fast facts. June 2004. Available at: www.nof.org/osteoporosis/stats.htm. Accessed July 24, 2004.

[5] Vargas CM, Kramarow EA, Yellowitz JA. The oral health of older Americans. Aging trends, No. 3. Hyattsville (MD): National Center for Health Statistics; 2001.

[6] Anonymous. Consensus development conference: diagnosis, prophylaxis, and treatment of osteoporosis. Am J Med 1993;94(6):646–50.

[7] Rosen CJ. Anatomy, physiology and disease. In: Langton CM, Njeh CF, editors. The physical measurement of bone. Bristol (UK): Institute of Physics Publishing; 2004. p. 20–1.

[8] Timiras PS. Aging of the skeleton, joints and muscles. In: Timiras PS, editor. Physiological basis of aging and geriatrics. 2nd edition. Boca Raton (FL): CRC Press; 1994. p. 259–72.

[9] US Preventive Services Task Force. Screening for osteoporosis in postmenopausal women: recommendations and rationale. Rockville (MD): Agency for Healthcare Research and Quality; September 2002. Available at: http://www.ahrq.gov/clinic/3rduspstf/osteoporosis/osteorr.htm. Accessed July 3, 2004.

[10] Njeh CF, Shepherd JA. Absorptiometric measurement. In: Langton CM, Njeh CF, editors. The physical measurement of bone. Bristol (UK): Institute of Physics Publishing; 2004. p. 267–307.

[11] Njeh CF, Shepherd J, Genant HK. Human studies. In: Langton CM, Njeh CF, editors. The physical measurement of bone. Bristol (UK): Institute of Physics Publishing; 2004. p. 551–70.

[12] World Health Organization. Assessment of fracture risk and its application to screening for postmenopausal osteoporosis. Geneva (Switzerland): World Health Organization; 1994. Technical Report Series No. 843. Available at: www.radiology.ab.ca/rcalinksOD.htm. Accessed August 12, 2004.

[13] National Osteoporosis Foundation. Physician's guide to prevention and treatment of osteoporosis. Washington, DC: National Osteoporosis Foundation; 2003 Available at: http://www.nof.org/physguide/pharmacologic.htm. Accessed August 12, 2004.

[14] NIH Consensus Development Panel. Osteoporosis prevention, diagnosis and therapy. JAMA 2001;285(6):785–95.

[15] Michaelsson K, Bergstrom R, Mallmin H, et al. Screening for osteopenia and osteoporosis: selection by body composition. Osteoporos Int 1996;6(2):120–6.

[16] Cadarette SM, Jaglal SB, Kreiger N, et al. Development and validation of the Osteoporosis Risk Assessment Instrument to facilitate selection of women for bone densitometry. CMAJ 2000;162(9):1289–94.

[17] Lydick E, Cook K, Turpin J, et al. Development and validation of a simple questionnaire to facilitate identification of women likely to have low bone density. Am J Manag Care 1998; 4(1):37–48.

[18] Reginster J-Y. A simple clinical tool that included age, weight, and estrogen use helped to select women for bone densitometry. ACP J Club 2001;134(1):37.

[19] National Institutes of Health. Optimal calcium intake. NIH Consensus Statement Online 1994(June 6–8);12(4):1–31. Available at: http://consensus.nih.gov/cons/097_statement.htm. Accessed August 11, 2004.

[20] National Institutes of Health. Osteoporosis overview fact sheets. Bethesda (MD): NIH Osteoporosis and Related Bone Diseases National Resources Center; 2003 Available at: www.osteo.org/newfile.asp?doc = osteo&doctitle = Osteoporosis+Overview&doctype = HTML+Fact+Sheet. Accessed August 12, 2004.

[21] Rosen CJ. Nutrition and bone health in the elderly. In: Holick MF, Dawson-Hughes B, editors. Nutrition and bone health. Totowa (NJ): Humana Press; 2004. p. 211–26.

[22] Dawson-Hughes B. Calcium and vitamin D for bone health in adults. In: Holick MF, Dawson-Hughes B, editors. Nutrition and bone health. Totowa (NJ): Humana Press; 2004. p. 197–210.

[23] Timiras ML. The skin and connective tissue. In: Timiras PS, editor. Physiological basis of aging and geriatrics. Boca Raton (FL): CRC Press; 1994. p. 273–8.

[24] Lipschitz DA. Nutrition. In: Cassel CK, Leipzig RM, Cohen HJ, et al, editors. Geriatric medicine: an evidence based approach. 4th edition. New York: Springer-Verlag; 2003. p. 1009–21.

[25] Krall EA, Wehler C, Garcia RI, et al. Calcium and vitamin D supplements reduce tooth loss in the elderly. Am J Med 2001;111(6):452–6.

[26] Department of Health and Human Services, Centers for Disease Control and Prevention, National Center for Chronic Disease Prevention and Health Promotion, Office on Smoking and Health. The health consequences of smoking: a report of the Surgeon General [Atlanta, GA]. Washington, DC: 2004. Available at: http://www.cdc.gov/tobacco/sgr/sgr_2004/chapters.htm. Accessed August 13, 2004.

[27] Kiel DP. Smoking, alcohol and bone health. In: Holick MF, Dawson-Hughes B, editors. Nutrition and bone health. Totowa (NJ): Humana Press; 2004. p. 481–513.

[28] Law M. Smoking and osteoporosis. In: Wald N, Baron J, editors. Smoking and hormone related disorders. New York: Oxford University Press; 1990. p. 83–92.

[29] Scane AC, Francis RM, Sutcliffe AM, et al. Case-controlled study of the pathogenesis and sequelae of symptomatic vertebral fractures in men. Osteoporos Int 1999;9(1):91–7.

[30] Jacqmin-Gadda H, Fourrier A, Commenges D, et al. Risk factors for fractures in the elderly. Epidemiology 1998;9(4):417–23.

[31] Heaney RP. Effects of caffeine on bone and the calcium economy. Food Chem Toxicol 2002; 40(9):1263–70.

[32] Rapuri PB, Gallagher JC, Kinyamu HK, et al. Caffeine intake increases the rate of bone loss in elderly women and interacts with vitamin D receptor genotypes. Am J Clin Nutr 2001; 74(5):694–700.

[33] Macdonald HM, New SA, Golden MH, et al. Nutritional associations with bone loss during the menopausal transition: evidence of a beneficial effect of calcium, alcohol, and fruit and vegetable nutrients and of a detrimental effect of fatty acids. Am J Clin Nutr 2004;79(1): 155–65.

[34] Feskanich D, Korrick SA, Greenspan SL, et al. Moderate alcohol consumption and bone density among postmenopausal women. J Womens Health 1999;8:65–73.

[35] Gong Z, Wezeman FH. Inhibitory effect of alcohol on osteogenic differentiation in human bone marrow–derived mesenchymal stem cells. Alcohol Clin Exp Res 2004;28(3):468–79.

[36] Kim MJ, Shim MS, Kim MK, et al. Effect of chronic alcohol ingestion on bone mineral density in males without liver cirrhosis. Korean J Intern Med 2003;18(3):174–80.

[37] Inzerillo A, Iqbal J, Troen B, et al. Skeletal fragility in the elderly. In: Cassel CK, Leipzig RM, Cohen HJ, et al, editors. Geriatric medicine: an evidence based approach. 4th edition. New York: Springer-Verlag; 2003. p. 621–50.

[38] Bloom H. Prevention. In: Cassel CK, Leipzig RM, Cohen HJ, et al, editors. Geriatric medicine: an evidence based approach. 4th edition. New York: Springer-Verlag; 2003. p. 169–84.

[39] Krall EA, Garcia RI, Dawson-Hughes B. Increased risk of tooth loss is related to bone loss at the whole body, hip, and spine. Calcif Tissue Int 1996;59(6):433–7.

[40] August M, Chung K, Chang YC, et al. Influence of estrogen status and endosseous implant osseointegration. J Oral Maxillofac Surg 2001;59:1285–91.

[41] Jeffcoat M. Osteoporosis: a possible modifying factor in oral bone loss. Ann Periodontol 1998;3:312–21.

[42] Gage TW, Pickett FA. Dental drug reference. 6th edition. St Louis (MO): Mosby; 2003.

[43] Watts NB. Bisphosphonates for treatment of osteoporosis. In: Favus MJ, editor. Primer on the metabolic bone diseases and disorders of mineral metabolism. 5th edition. Washington, DC: American Society for Bone and Mineral Research; 2003. p. 338–9.

[44] Delmas PD. Clinical use of selective estrogen receptor modulators and other estrogen analogs. In: Favus MJ, editor. Primer on the metabolic bone diseases and disorders of mineral metabolism. 5th edition. Washington, DC: American Society for Bone and Mineral Research; 2003. p. 331–5.

[45] Ke HZ, Qi H, Chidsey-Frink KL, et al. Lasofoxifene (CP-336, 156) protects against the age-related changes in bone mass, bone strength, and total serum cholesterol in intact aged male rats. J Bone Miner Res 2001;16:765–73.

[46] Bjarnason NH, Bjarnason K, Haarbo J, et al. Tibolone: prevention of bone loss in late postmenopausal women. J Clin Endocrinol Metab 1996;81:2419–22.

[47] Berning B, Kuijk CV, Kuiper JW, et al. Effects of two doses of tibolone on trabecular and cortical bone loss in early postmenopausal women: a two-year randomized, placebo-controlled study. Bone 1996;19:395–9.

[48] Harvard Health Publications Newsletter. April 2004. Available at: http://www.health.harvard.edu/hhp/article/content.do?name = W1201c. Accessed August 8, 2004.

[49] Watts NB. Pharmacology of agents to treat osteoporosis. In: Favus MJ, editor. Primer on the metabolic bone diseases and disorders of mineral metabolism. 4th edition. Philadelphia: Lippincott Williams & Wilkins; 1999. p. 278–83.

[50] Dawson-Hughes B. Pharmacologic treatment of postmenopausal osteoporosis. In: Favus MJ, editor. Primer on the metabolic bone diseases and disorders of mineral metabolism. 4th edition. Philadelphia: Lippincott Williams & Wilkins; 1999. p. 283–8.

[51] Ringe JD. Fluoride and bone health. In: Holick MF, Dawson-Hughes B, editors. Nutrition and bone health. Totowa (NJ): Humana Press; 2004. p. 345–62.

[52] Ringe JD, Kipshoven C, Coster A, et al. Therapy of established postmenopausal osteoporosis and monofluorophosphate plus calcium: dose-related effects on bone density and fracture rate. Osteoporos Int 1999;9(2):171–8.

[53] Reeve J. Teriparatide (rhPTH[1–34]) and future anabolic treatments for osteoporosis. In: Favus MJ, editor. Primer on the metabolic bone diseases and disorders of mineral metabolism. 5th edition. Washington, DC: American Society for Bone and Mineral Research; 2003. p. 344–8.

[54] Mundy G, Garrett R, Harris S, et al. Stimulation of bone formation in vitro and in rodents by statins. Science 1999;286:1946–9.

[55] Meraw SJ, Reeve CM, Wollan PC. Use of alendronate in peri-implant defect regeneration. J Periodontol 1999;70(2):151–8.

[56] Denissen H, Montanari C, Martinetti R, et al. Alveolar bone response to submerged bisphosphonate-complexed hydroxyapatite implants. J Periodontol 2000;71(2):279–86.

[57] Kaynak D, Meffert R, Bostanci H, et al. A histopathological investigation on the effect of systemic administration of the bisphosphonate alendronate on resorptive phase following mucoperiosteal flap surgery in the rat mandible. J Periodontol 2003;74(9):1348–54.

[58] Demerjian N, Bolla G, Spreux A. Severe oral ulcerations induced by alendronate. Clin Rheumatol 1999;18(4):349–50.

[59] Ruggiero SL, Mehrotra B, Rosenberg TJ, et al. Osteonecrosis of the jaws associated with the use of bisphosphonates: a review of 63 cases. J Oral Maxillofac Surg 2004;62(5): 527–34.

[60] El-Shinnawi UM, El-Tantawy SI. The effect of alendronate sodium on alveolar bone loss in periodontitis (clinical trial). J Int Acad Periodontol 2003;5(1):5–10.

[61] Reddy MS, Geurs NC, Gunsolley JC. Periodontal host modulation with antiproteinase, anti-inflammatory and bone-sparing agents. A systemic review. Ann Periodontol 2003;8(1): 12–37.

[62] Orwoll ES. Osteoporosis in men. In: Favus MJ, editor. Primer on the metabolic bone diseases and disorders of mineral metabolism. 5th edition. Washington, DC: American Society for Bone and Mineral Research; 2003. p. 361–3.

[63] Orwoll ES. The prevention and therapy of osteoporosis in men. In: Orwoll ES, editor. Osteoporosis in men. San Diego (CA): Academic Press; 1999. p. 562–3.

[64] Wactawski-Wende J. Oral bone loss and osteoporosis. In: Favus MJ, editor. Primer on the metabolic bone diseases and disorders of mineral metabolism. 5th edition. Washington, DC: American Society for Bone and Mineral Research; 2003. p. 541–4.

[65] Zeeman GG, Veth EO, Dennison DK. Focus on primary care: periodontal disease: implications for women's health. Obstet Gynecol Surv 2001;56(1):43–9.

[66] Von Wowern N. In vivo measurement of bone mineral content of mandibles by dual-photon absorptiometry. Scand J Dent Res 1985;93:162–8.

484 MULLIGAN & SOBEL

[67] Von Wowern N, Storm TL, Olgaard K. Bone mineral content by photon absorptiometry of the mandible compared with that of the forearm and the lumbar spine. Calcif Tissue Int 1988; 42:157–61.

[68] Corten FG, van't Hof MA, Buijs WC, et al. Measurement of mandibular bone density ex vivo and in vivo by dual energy absorptiometry. Arch Oral Biol 1993;38(3):215–9.

[69] Horner K, Devlin H, Alsop CW, et al. Mandibular bone mineral density as a predictor of skeletal osteoporosis. Br J Radiol 1996;69(827):1019–25.

[70] Devlin H, Horner K, Ledgerton D. A comparison of maxillary and mandibular bone mineral densities. J Prosthet Dent 1998;79:323–7.

[71] Horner K, Devlin H. The relationship between two indices of mandibular bone quality and bone mineral density measured by dual energy x-ray absorptiometry. Dentomaxillofac Radiol 1998;27(1):17–21.

[72] Kribbs P, Chesnut C. Relationships between mandibular and skeletal bone in an osteoporotic population. J Prosthet Dent 1989;62:703–7.

[73] Jonasson G, Bankvall G, Kiliaridis S. Estimation of skeletal bone mineral density by means of the trabecular pattern of the alveolar bone, its interdental thickness, and the bone mass of the mandible. Oral Surg Oral Med Oral Pathol Oral Radiol Endod 2001;92:346–52.

[74] Sanfilippo F, Bianchi AE. Osteoporosis: the effect on maxillary bone resorption and therapeutic possibilities by means of implant prostheses—a literature review and clinical considerations. Int J Periodontics Restorative Dent 2003;23(5):447–57.

[75] Bianchi A, Sanfilippo F. Osteoporosis: the effect on mandibular bone resorption and therapeutic possibilities by means of implant prostheses. Int J Periodontics Restorative Dent 2002;22(3):230–9.

[76] Hirai T, Ishijima T, Hashikawa Y, et al. Osteoporosis and reduction of residual ridge in edentulous patients. J Prosthet Dent 1993;69:49–56.

[77] Klemetti E. A review of residual ridge resorption and bone density. J Prosthet Dent 1996; 75(5):512–4.

[78] Southard KA, Southard TE, Schlechte JA, et al. The relationship between the density of the alveolar processes and that of post-cranial bone. J Dent Res 2000;79(4):964–9.

[79] Becker W, Hujoel PP, Becker BE, et al. Osteoporosis and implant failure: an exploratory case-control study. J Periodontol 2000;71(4):625–31.

[80] van Steenberghe D, Jacobs R, Desnyder M, et al. The relative impact of local and endogenous patient-related factors on implant failure up to the abutment stage. Clin Oral Implants Res 2002;13(6):617–22.

[81] Friberg B, Ekestubbe A, Mellstrom D, et al. Branemark implants and osteoporosis: a clinical exploratory study. Clin Implant Dent Relat Res 2001;3(1):50–6.

[82] von Wowern N. General and oral aspects of osteoporosis: a review. Clin Oral Invest 2001; 5(2):71–82.

[83] National Osteoporosis Foundation. Advocacy news and updates. Available at: http://www.nof.org/advocacy/prevalence/index.htm. Accessed July 24, 2004.

[84] Boonen S, Rizzoli R, Meunier PJ, et al. The need for clinical guidance in the use of calcium and vitamin D in the management of osteoporosis: a consensus report. Osteoporos Int 2004; 15(7):511–9.

ELSEVIER
SAUNDERS

THE DENTAL
CLINICS
OF NORTH AMERICA

Dent Clin N Am 49 (2005) 485–490

Index

Note: Page numbers of article titles are in **boldface** type.

0011-8532/05/$ - see front matter © 2005 Elsevier Inc. All rights reserved.
doi:10.1016/S0011-8532(05)00013-3   *dental.theclinics.com*